ALL IN A DOCTOR'S DAY

Dr Lucia Gannon qualified as a general practitioner in 1990. She has special interests in mental health, infant nutrition and medical education. She is an Assistant Programme Director with the South East GP Training Scheme and was a GP Clinical Tutor for University of Limerick Graduate Entry Medical School (GEMS) from 2010 to 2018, and works with her husband at Killenaule Surgery, Co. Tipperary.

ALL IN A DOCTOR'S DAY

MEMOIRS OF AN IRISH COUNTRY PRACTICE

Dr Lucia Gannon

Gill Books

Gill Books

Hume Avenue

Park West

Dublin 12

www.gillbooks.ie

Gill Books is an imprint of M.H. Gill and Co.

© Lucia Gannon 2019

978 07171 8325 8

Design and print origination by O'K Graphic Design, Dublin

Edited by Alison Walsh

Proofread by Jane Rogers

Printed by CPI Group (UK) Ltd, Croydon CRO 4YY

This book is typeset in 12.5/17 pt Minion.

The paper used in this book comes from the wood pulp of managed forests. For every tree felled, at least one tree is planted, thereby renewing natural resources.

Text from the introduction to this book first appeared in an article in the *Medical Independent* called 'The Art of Gracious Acceptance'

In order to protect patient confidentiality, many patient details, including age, gender and life circumstances have been altered. Many of the characters are an amalgam of two or three people. However, the people, life situations and dilemmas described do represent my experience of over twenty years of general practice. All dialogue is an imprecise recollection of conversations and consultations that I hope captures the essence of the doctor–patient interaction and conveys the thoughts and feelings that I experience as I go about my daily work. All family and friends are real people in my life.

ACKNOWLEDGEMENTS

I would like to thank all at Gill, especially Deirdre, who inspired me to write this book and who encouraged and supported me through the process. Also Sheila and Alison, whose editorial expertise nudged the submitted draft to what it is today.

Priscilla, Catherine and Paul, at *Medical Independent*, for publishing my first columns and convincing me that not only had I something to say, but that people enjoyed reading them. All the readers of those columns who have given me positive feedback over the years.

Special thanks to Irene Graham, Story Editor and founder of *The Creative Writer's Workshop* and *The Memoir Writing Club*. Her expertise, encouragement and patience were invaluable at every stage of the process.

To my friends and fellow book club members, Judith, Dolores, Ann, Heather, Marie Therese, Jacinta, Kate, Cora and Anne, who have for years encouraged me to write a book, continuously checked on my progress and provided timely distractions when needed.

All the patients who have trusted me with their stories and brought humour, wisdom and kindness to my life. All who have worked in Killenaule Surgery over the years: Noreen, Bridget, Elaine, Angela, Siobhan, Marissa, AnneMarie, Delia, Bernie, Grace, Maggie, Wally and Pat. The GPs in our neighbouring districts, John, Carmel and Molly, who were always on-hand to help out when needed. Denise, Leanne, Angela and Therese, who looked after my children as if they were their own.

My three children, Joseph, Ailshe and Liam Jnr, for their enthusiasm and trust as I wrote the details of their lives. And finally, my husband, Liam, a bottomless well of love, encouragement, patience and support, and without whom none of this would have been possible.

To my father and step-mother, Paddy and Mary Gannon,
for their unwavering love and support.

To the memory of my birth mother, Teresa (Tessie) Gannon,
whose untimely death left me with a greater appreciation of life
and who, despite her absence, was always present.

CONTENTS

WITH GRACIOUS ACCEPTANCE

'I washed my windows yesterday,' she said.

'Oh, my goodness,' I replied, 'You must be feeling well.'

'I am, thank God,' she said with a smile. 'Every day I get up early, do a bit of housework, take a stroll around the garden; if it's dry, I call to my neighbour for a chat and listen to a bit of local radio, just to keep in touch with what is going on. I like to get the death notices,' she went on in the same cheerful tone, 'I don't like not to know if someone has died. At my age, I know more of those in the departure than the arrival lounge, I'm afraid.'

There was nothing morose about her words, no regret or self-pity. Just acceptance and gratitude for the life she had and the fact that she was still here, while many were not. I was waiting for her prescription to print, standing over the printer to pre-empt a paper jam. (I have deliberately placed the printer as far away as possible from my chair, so that I have to get up and walk over to it every time I print something; a combination of maintaining circulation to the extremities and subconsciously signalling the close of the consultation.) Looking across at her, I found myself hoping that I would grow old like this woman. There was something serene and joyful about her. I wondered if I should share this insight with her. I decided not to. I was already behind with appointments and needed to move on.

She looked at me as if she knew I was going to say something and had changed my mind. I sat back down alongside her, head bent over the script, while signing it. 'I haven't seen you for a while,' she said, 'it was your husband I met the last few times. I was a bit worried that you might not be well.'

I looked up and saw the concern on her face. 'Oh, not at all, not a bother on me, thankfully,' I replied, 'I must have been off gallivanting.'

'Oh, good,' she answered. 'My neighbour said she had been in to you, so I figured that was it.'

I relaxed my pose and decided that although the consultation might be complete, life was too short not to engage a little longer. 'It's very kind of you to think of me,' I said. 'I do appreciate your concern.'

'Oh, you have a hard job, Doctor, and I don't know how you do it, day after day, sitting here listening to the likes of me and taking care of sick people all the time. I often think of you and your family and say a prayer that ye will all have good health.'

I wondered who was caring for who in this complicated human interaction: me, the doctor in my consulting seat, my mind already on the next patient, or this elderly lady, over thirty years my senior, letting me know that I was not just a doctor, but that I mattered to her and that she remembered me and my family in her prayers. I was humbled. With a start, I realised that I could have missed this, a precious gift of caring and kindness, offered unbidden with no strings attached. I could have gone automatically through my day and denied myself the love, gratitude and concern that this lady was offering.

She rose, took her script from my outstretched hand and made her way to the door. 'Goodbye, now, Doctor,' she said. 'It was good to see you.'

'And you,' I replied, holding open the door and touching her lightly on the shoulder as she went out.

Within a week she was gone. Slipped away quietly in her sleep, it appeared. Her neighbour found her the next day when she did not arrive for her usual chat. It did not surprise me. Despite her apparent good health, she had a number of illnesses, all gently but stealthily stealing her breath, leading steadfastly to her last.

Medicine has limits, but kindness does not. I learned a lesson from this beautiful lady and am grateful that I did. People are the reason I do my job. These people I meet every day come with gifts of compassion, kindness, gratitude, wisdom and love. I just need to allow myself to receive them.

I didn't get to hear her name announced on the death notices, but I did call to her house a couple of days later to pay my respects. There, sticking out from the mantelpiece, was the prescription I had given her the week before. Later, in the surgery, I checked her file and discovered that it wasn't actually due for renewal for a further three weeks. I wondered if she had felt that her end was near and had come to say goodbye.

General practitioners provide care for all individuals, regardless of age, sex or illness: they include physical, psychological and social factors in their decision-making; use repeated contacts to gather information; gain the trust of those they serve while maintaining a professional role in the community. I have tried to do those things and more since I came to Killenaule to work as a GP more than twenty years ago. I have maintained my clinical skills so that I can attend to medical emergencies, manage chronic disease, diagnose childhood illnesses and provide antenatal and terminal care; I have learned to sit in relative calm, knowing a storm is coming, when I see the first signs of frailty, the beginnings of failing memory or the insidious onset of depression. In doing this, I have come to know and trust the people I care for, as they have come to know and trust me.

The consultation is at the heart of all general practice. In the privacy of my consulting room, with my eyes, ears and mind finely tuned to the patient, I do my most difficult work, but this is also where I receive my greatest rewards. As a surgeon might experience a high after completing a particularly complicated operation, I, too, can feel elated and energised after completing a particularly complex consultation. A consultation where I have listened to a patient's story, helped them make sense of the narrative, distinguished between disease and distress and negotiated a way forward, while guarding against unnecessary interventions. At other times, I have simply been present as a witness to their suffering. During these interactions, it is as if time stands still as I am fully engaged, balanced on the edge of my competence, with a definite goal: that of making sure that this patient feels heard and understood, that they experience compassion, even if they do not recognise it as such.

I am grateful to all the patients who have trusted me with their stories and who have enriched my life with their presence – far too many to write about. For the purposes of confidentiality, it has been necessary to alter the names and many of the details of the patients who appear in this book, but while the people are altered, the sentiments remain the same. The many lessons I have learned are real and have made me the doctor that I am. As with all memories, my story is subject to bias and the altered perspective that comes with retrospection, but while writing this book, I have tried to depict as accurately as possible the joys and the sorrows, the challenges and the rewards of being an Irish country GP.

CHAPTER ONE

THE BEST-LAID PLANS

One dark Sunday in February 1998, I slipped out of bed and made my way to the bathroom across the hall. At thirty-eight weeks pregnant, this had become a frequent nocturnal activity, one that I could almost carry out in my sleep, but that night, or morning – it was too dark to tell – I was wide awake. My baby's kicking and wriggling had woken me, as if suggesting that it was no longer happy within that cramped space. I had no pain and no contractions, but at that moment I realised that my waters had broken and that my intuition was right. My baby did need to be born.

In the dim bathroom light, I stared at my reflection in the mirror. A tired, drawn and pale face stared back. 'I know this is not what you had planned for today,' I said to my reflection, in as kind and reassuring a voice as I could muster, 'but by this evening you will have your baby. And everything will be alright.' I was officially on maternity leave from the busy GP practice that I shared with my husband, Liam, and was looking forward to the birth of our third child. I placed my hand on my swollen abdomen and spoke just as softly to my baby. 'You'll be out soon. Just another couple of hours.'

Just then, I heard the house telephone ring in the bedroom. My husband's sleepy voice answered it. 'Yes, this is Doctor Meagher,' he said. 'Who am I speaking to?'

The rest of the house was silent apart from the odd creak of timber and the rain that had started to fall on the Velux window over my head. Further down the hall, our two children, Joseph and Ailshe, were still asleep. I resisted the urge to go to their rooms and check on them. We would have to wake them soon enough. I knew what I needed: I needed whoever was on the phone to stop talking, I needed someone to mind my children and I needed Liam to get me to the hospital.

When I re-entered the bedroom Liam was sitting up in bed. 'Have you tried your own doctor?' he was saying into the phone, rolling his eyes and giving me an apologetic look. 'OK, OK. I understand. If you really think you need to be seen early, come to the house at about eight-thirty, before I leave to start the morning surgery. I will see you then.'

I slipped back into bed. It was not yet six o'clock on that dark and windy February morning. I waited for Liam to finish his conversation, trying to formulate a plan for the day. Liam sat back against the pillows and sighed deeply, covering the mouthpiece with his hand, while still listening. Whatever the person on the other end was saying, I could tell that they were being pretty insistent.

'OK,' Liam said, with an undisguised air of resignation. 'Just let me take down the directions and I will be out as soon as I can.'

I tapped him on the shoulder. Pointing at my swollen belly, I shook my head and mouthed a silent 'hospital'.

He gave me a puzzled look. My baby was to be born by planned caesarean section the following day, Tuesday, 10 February, the same birthday as my grandmother, not Monday, 9 February. For a split second, Liam looked as if he was about to remind me of this and point out that I had mixed up my dates, but then swiftly changed his mind. I was not one to raise false alarms. He turned his attention back to the phone. 'I'm very sorry,' he said. 'From what you have told me so far, you do not need a doctor right now. You can call your own doctor later and arrange to see him. I'm afraid my wife is in labour and I need to get her to the hospital.'

I had never heard him speak so firmly to a patient, especially someone he did not know, but there was no way either of us could see a patient that morning: they would all have to wait for another day, see another doctor, or go to the hospital. We did not have a replacement doctor for the surgery for emergency situations such as this, nor did I have a doctor to replace me while I was on leave, which is why I had continued to see a reduced number of patients until two days earlier, when I'd finally decided to leave my consulting room and not return until after my baby was born and I felt well enough to do so. I knew our colleagues in the neighbouring villages of Ballingarry and Fethard were aware of our situation and were on standby to see any patients who needed attention. That was the only emergency plan we had.

Liam had told a white lie to the person at the other end of the telephone: I was not actually in labour, but I needed to get to the hospital without delay, because my baby was breech. For the last four months of pregnancy, my son (although I did not know at that time whether I would give birth to a boy or a girl) had positioned himself with his head nestled under my ribs and nothing I could say or do would persuade him to turn himself around. That was the reason for the planned caesarean section, but because the fluid that protects the baby was draining away, there was a risk of his umbilical cord becoming squashed against the muscular wall of the womb, depriving him of oxygen, so the section could not be delayed.

Both Liam and I knew the risks associated with a breech delivery. We had both worked in obstetrics and paediatrics during our GP training in the UK and had intubated and resuscitated perfectly formed, healthy-looking babies, who had become deprived of oxygen during such a delivery. And of course, all doctors know that medical people make the worst patients, that they attract complications like electrons to protons, the negative to the positive, or, at least, that is the common perception. That morning, all these possibilities remained present but unspoken. However, they were not fears – they were merely facts. We had been blessed with two healthy children and were both confident that this time would be the same.

My bag was packed, there was petrol in the car, but the previous night my childminder had called to say that she was ill and would not be back to work for the foreseeable future. I needed a plan before I woke Ailshe and Joseph from their slumber, where they remained, as yet unaware of the impending disturbance to their routine. Coming up with such a plan was not easy. Liam and I had only been living in Killenaule for a couple of years, since we had taken on the GP practice. We did not have a network of people whom we could call on in emergency situations, but I had made one friend and it was to her that my thoughts turned at that time.

Judith and I had crossed paths one day about a year earlier, as she was manoeuvring her toddler son and three-year-old daughter out of the local shop. It might have been her Northern Irish accent, which singled her out as another person who did not fully belong in this South Tipperary village, that drew me to her. It might have been that her bright and chatty daughter, Gráinne, was the same age as Ailshe and went to the same playschool in the neighbouring town of Fethard, or it may have been that the light blue summer sundress she was wearing that day, as she and her children enjoyed messy ice-cream cones, gave her a carefree air, making me sense that this was a person at ease in the world, with the capacity to find joy in the ordinary. As luck would have it, I was walking in her direction and we fell into easy conversation, two blow-in, migrant mothers, tentatively putting down roots in what we hoped was fertile soil. Before we parted, we had already made arrangements to meet again and so we embarked on a friendship that would enhance many a high point, sustain me through many a crisis and accompany me on a path that would have appeared dull and lacklustre without her. However, even though all of that was still to come, I knew, at that early stage, that I could count on her, even if, as now, it was only six o'clock in the morning and she was not expecting a call from me.

Ailshe appeared at the bedroom door, a sleepy four-year-old who knew, even in a house where phones rang and children migrated in and out of beds at all hours of the night, that morning was a bit more active than usual.

'I'm afraid I have to go to the hospital today and not tomorrow,' I said. Ailshe was a girl who did not like surprises, especially if they entailed separation from her mother. I was rarely parted from herself and Joseph, and as I knew this separation would be for more than a few nights, I had prepared them both as best I could. One afternoon, a few weeks earlier, I had asked them what they would miss most when I was away. Almost immediately they had both replied that it would be my bedtime reading. The next day we had picked out some of their favourite books, and in the following weeks, while I had rested in the afternoons, too tired and slow to do anything else, I had recorded myself reading as many excerpts as I could on an old-fashioned cassette recorder. It was no hardship for me. I did not need an excuse to read, especially when the books they had picked included *The Secret Garden, Watership Down* and other classics that I was only discovering as an adult.

Despite suggestions from well-meaning friends and relatives that my children were 'too attached', that I was causing them to become too dependent on me, I did not believe that, as I could observe the signs of their developing independence. Besides, I believed that it was easier to set sail from a safe harbour than to try to begin a journey on a stormy sea and I tried to provide this harbour while I could. At least, that was what I hoped I was doing. That was what the books I chose to read would have me believe I was doing: Rosalind Miles's *The Children We Deserve*, D.W. Winnicott's *Home is Where We Start From*, and Penelope Leach's *Children First*, are just some of the well-thumbed volumes that still line my bookshelves, mementoes of early motherhood and my striving to do the right thing. Of course, I only read what I wanted to hear and avoided any self-professed expert or guru who might recommend strict schedules, exacting routines or separation from my children.

'Your voice sounds funny,' Ailshe had said when I had played some of the cassette back to her, 'but I still know it is you.' I reminded her now that she could listen to these stories any time she liked and that before she knew it, I would be back home with a new baby brother or sister. She dressed herself in an orange skirt and purple top of her own choosing, indicating to me that she was ready to face the day.

Joseph followed, also fully dressed, his face a mixture of concern and anticipation. At six years of age, he already carried the responsibility of being the eldest child. With him, I had made more mistakes, struggled with more uncertainties and worried more about doing things exactly right, but it was also with him that I had first experienced that overwhelming love for my own child and a realisation that my life would never be the same again. As he left for Judith's home with his dad and his sister, his schoolbag over one shoulder, a box of Weetabix tucked under his other arm, I reminded myself that despite his mature and confident demeanour, he would not be fully convinced that all was well in the world until I was back home again.

Fifteen minutes later, they returned. 'The Fennellys are all either drugged or dead,' Liam said, referring to Judith and her family, when he came back with Joseph and Ailshe trailing behind him, looking forlorn and worried. 'I have been ringing and ringing and pounding on the door, but there is not a stir from inside. Even though both cars are in the yard.'

I did not know how anyone could sleep so soundly. I seemed to hear every leaf falling and every branch creaking throughout the night and woke with the slightest provocation. I assumed it was from years of broken sleep as a junior doctor. I knew Liam would have done all he could to wake them: unlike me, he knew when to ask for help and did not consider it a personal failure to do so.

'I'm afraid ye will just have to come with us,' Liam said to the two worried faces. 'They might let ye wait in the hospital foyer and then come up to see the baby before I bring ye back home. Ye might even be back in time for school,' he joked.

I wasn't in the mood for humour. Then I remembered that about a week earlier, while I'd waited for Joseph at the school gate, a mother called Deirdre had offered to do the school run and to help out with the kids anytime if I was stuck. I appreciated her kindness and knew her offer was genuine so I'd thanked her and said I would keep her in mind, never thinking that I would have to take her up on her offer. Now, I reminded Liam about that offer, adding that I really did not like to impose on her.

'She wouldn't have offered if she didn't mean it,' Liam replied, in his usual matter-of-fact manner, and without further discussion, without consideration of the 'coulds' or 'shoulds', he turned to the kids. 'OK, guys, let's go again. As usual, Mum has another plan.'

When he returned, almost half an hour later, he was alone and looked relieved. 'You would think she was expecting them,' he said. 'No problem at all. I didn't even need to explain: she just took them in and told me I'd better get going.

Getting to the hospital was the easiest problem to solve that morning, and once we did, our baby, Liam Junior, was born, pink and healthy, weighing over eight pounds. I was alive and well, if a bit stiff and sore. As soon as I could, I put him to my breast and he suckled as if he knew instinctively that his life depended on it. I had breastfed both Joseph and Ailshe well into toddlerhood. This was not a common practice in Ireland in the early 90s, when Joseph was born, and while it was probably a little more acceptable in theory in 1998, there were still lots of people who felt uncomfortable with the idea that babies were breastfed, especially babies over six months of age, so it was not something I advertised although I did not deny it or try to justify it.

Even as a qualified GP who had worked extensively in obstetrics and paediatrics, I had had no knowledge of breastfeeding when I had my first baby. It was not a topic that was included in textbooks or lectures and in the hospitals in which I'd worked in the UK, during my four years of GP training, I rarely saw mothers breastfeeding successfully. The calls I would get from the postnatal ward were usually from experienced midwives, who informed me that the mothers were having difficulty, that they did not have enough milk and that the babies were hungry. I was usually asked to give my imprimatur to a 'top-up' of formula milk, to help them over this hump. Not knowing any better, I took my cue from them and gave it. I did not know at the time that this was the worst thing I could have done, that a single top-up feed could result in the end of the breastfeeding relationship for these mothers and babies and that what they needed was encouragement and support from someone with knowledge of the breastfeeding process. I only learned that later, when I had my own children. This had been a steep learning curve for me, but once I was convinced that breastfeeding was the best thing to do, I was determined to succeed.

In those pre-internet and pre-Amazon days, finding relevant information was a challenge, but I was fortunate to discover a copy of Sheila Kitzinger's *The Experience of Breastfeeding* in a small bookshop, a book that opened the door to a very different way of mothering and childcare than what I had been exposed to as a junior doctor. Armed with this new knowledge, I became my own expert, so that by the time I gave birth to Liam Jnr, I was determined not to let anyone endanger my breastfeeding efforts. While in hospital with my new baby, I guarded him with the tenacity of a lioness, never letting him out of my sight and feeding him at every available opportunity, making sure that no one would give him a top-up. That was all I could do. I could not think about the fact that I would have no one to help me manage the house and the children when I got home: Liam had returned to work the day after Liam Jnr was born. He had no choice. It was not possible to find a replacement doctor and someone needed to provide care for our patients. I could not think about who would take care of me and my children. All of that would sort itself out, I hoped. I tried to convince myself that what mattered was that my baby was well and healthy. That we had another little miracle that should not be taken for granted.

Liam told me not to worry, that he would sort something out and I had to believe that he would. On the day after my caesarean section, I awoke from a nap to find two of my eight sisters, Marian and Treasa, sitting by my bed. 'We can stay a few days,' Marian said, 'so you needn't worry for now. And Liam just told us before we left that he might have found someone to mind the kids.'

I cried tears of relief in response to their kindness. As a doctor, I was not used to asking for help. I was usually the one offering it, but now, I let my sisters' concern envelop me. It felt nice, like a thick, warm fog that shielded me temporarily from the world – a world I had no wish to face just then.

Later that day I rang my home. A young woman answered the phone, and told me her name was Denise. I explained who I was and thanked her for coming to mind the children at such short notice. 'It's no bother,' she replied, as if she had known me all my life. I remember thinking that her voice sounded kind and confident and I tried to imagine what she looked like, but I was too tired and fell into an uneasy sleep. By the time I came home from hospital, Denise was well on the way to winning the affection of our two sceptical children. She seemed to instinctively understand Ailshe's need for planning and Joseph's preference to be left to do his own thing. With her help, order was restored: laundry was done, dinners were cooked and I got back to my bedtime reading routine. Only from then on, our reading group contained one extra pair of little ears.

As spring turned to summer, my thoughts returned to getting back to work and to the ever-increasing list that Bridget, the practice secretary, was compiling, the list of the people who wanted an appointment with the 'Lady Doctor', as soon as she was back from maternity leave.

CHAPTER TWO

'THE HILLS OF KILLENAULE'

At some point in the months after our youngest child's birth, Liam and Bridget moved to work in the new surgery that we had built on a greenfield site on the outskirts of the village. The move had been delayed due to difficulties in getting an electricity pole erected: I had given up asking Liam when it would happen, as he didn't have an answer. Eventually, it did happen, but there was no fanfare to mark the date, there were no politicians cutting ribbons, there was no cheese and wine reception with photographs for the local paper. Liam and Bridget simply left the Health Board premises they had been working in on a Friday evening, stuck a sign on the door saying, WE HAVE MOVED, loaded the patient files into the boot of Liam's car and transferred them to the new building, less than half a mile away. The following Monday morning they opened for business. We had not thought of a name for the new premises, so it became known as 'The Surgery,' to distinguish it from the old Health Board building, called 'The Clinic'. We were pleased with the architect-designed building, even if it did attract a lot of questions from locals as to why it was such an unusual shape. It had a curved wall facing the road that was not characteristic of doctor's surgeries or of any buildings in the locality.

'An architect!' Liam's father had exclaimed when we had first shown him the plans. 'I never heard of an architect designing a doctor's surgery.' He went on to say that he thought we were spending far too much money on building a new surgery and wondered why we could not stay in the one we were already in. I saw Liam's face fall as he folded up the plans and put them away. We had put a lot of thought into the design of the surgery and I knew Liam was proud of it. We would spend many hours in it, so the structure, the feel, the functionality of that space was just as important as the new house we intended to build higher up in the same field. We were renting the house that we lived in at that time and there were no suitable houses for sale in the village. (In those days, it was a condition of the medical-card contract that doctors reside in their practice area.) The surgery would be a place where people would come when they were ill, worried, confused and dying, where mothers would bring their new babies for routine checks and vaccinations, where toddlers would feel safe to come out from behind their mothers' or fathers' knees and allow us to place a stethoscope on their chests, or an auriscope in their ears. It would be a place where teenagers would talk freely and confidentially about acne, or anxiety, or contraception, a place where the old and frail would wait their turn in the comfort of a warm, bright waiting room. The Health Board premises that we had shared with the public health nurse, the dentist and the community welfare officer had a front door that would not stay closed, leading directly onto a corridor that doubled as a waiting room, with a floor that was constantly covered with the leaves and debris that had blown in from the street. The one consulting room that Liam and I had shared had no window, and barely enough room for an examination couch, a desk and two chairs. Staying there was not an option.

'I'm sorry your father was not more supportive or enthusiastic,' I said to Liam when we were alone later that night.

'I was a bit disappointed alright,' he said. 'But you know Dad. He just doesn't want us taking on too much financial responsibility and I think he still hopes that we might move again, a bit closer to Mam and himself in Galway.' Although Liam was originally from Mayo, his parents had moved to Galway just as Liam and I had finished medical school there and while we would like to have settled somewhere closer to them, at that time there were no opportunities for young GPs in Galway.

Liam's father was right, of course. Building a surgery was a big financial commitment, so his concern was understandable. We were also very unlikely to move again if we had invested in our own surgery, but I couldn't help but wish that he had kept his misgivings to himself. I wasn't always as slow to judge and as quick to forgive as Liam, qualities in him that have engendered equal measures of admiration and frustration in me over the years.

The finished building was modest and functional. It was wheelchair accessible with a bright, warm and spacious waiting area. The curved wall to the front encircled a large window that allowed light in, while at the same time protecting the privacy of the patients in the waiting room. We each had our own consulting room, with two extra rooms for a nurse, or a GP registrar, if we decided to become a teaching practice. Both Liam and I were interested in training GPs in Ireland. We had qualified as doctors from the National University of Ireland, Galway in 1986, at a time when training places for GPs were in short supply in Ireland, which was why we had both completed our GP training in the UK. We could see that Irish GPs were just as capable of providing good-quality training and wanted to be part of that process once we were established in our own practice.

The consulting room windows framed a view of Slievenamon, 'the mountain of the women', a heather-covered dome of a mountain steeped in legend and celebrated in song. It is said that Fionn mac Cumhaill had chosen his wife by picking the winner from a group of women who had run up that mountain. On a clear day, I could see the cairn on its summit, which reputedly marks the entrance to the Celtic underworld.

Patients congratulated us on our new building. Some brought potted plants or pictures for the walls. Some told their family and friends, who also came, slowly at first, to see what we were like. They laid out their problems like cases before the court, hoping for advice, or healing, or simply someone to accompany them on their journey. Those who did not like our image, our accent, our age, our appointment system or style of practice, took their problems elsewhere, to other doctors in the area, who, they felt, best suited their needs.

It had taken us two years to build the new surgery. Almost two years to the day since I had driven my children and myself in my grey Nissan Bluebird, stuffed with toys, clothes, books, nappies and anything else left over by the removal men, from the village of Drimoleague in West Cork to this village in South Tipperary in the shelter of the Slieveardagh foothills. It had been my second ever visit to Killenaule, the first having been about three months earlier for a brief look at the place where a practice had become available, due to the retirement of the previous GP, to see if we could make it our home. Liam had arrived a week earlier and had already rented a home for us to live in temporarily. The premises was situated on one of the main streets of Killenaule and on the day that I'd arrived, Liam was already at work.

As I pulled up outside the empty house, I accidentally drove too close to the footpath, which was separated from the road by a higher-than-usual kerb. With a thud, the underside of the car landed on the kerb, the inside wheels slipping onto the footpath. A passing garda would have been well within his rights to ask me to blow into a bag. There was no garda, but a man appeared from a nearby building, wiping his hands on a bloody butcher's apron. He surveyed the car, the footpath and me and then peered in to the back seat, at the two heads straining to see what all the fuss was about.

'Hello,' I said to the man, who, despite his intense interest in my predicament, did not appear very interested in conversation.

He looked at me again, a little closer this time. 'Are you the doctor's wife?' he asked.

I said I was and that I had just arrived and hoped I was in the right place. I also hoped he might have a suggestion as to how I could manoeuvre my car back onto the road before it became known that the doctor's wife could not park correctly. But I refrained from asking this. He said nothing in response, just disappeared into his shop, taking up his position inside the window, where he watched as I unloaded the car, while trying to keep a two-year-old and four-year-old from wandering on to the road. It wasn't such a great start.

Two years later, we were convinced that Killenaule was a good place to be. We still had to build a house, but we had each other, three healthy children and our very own new surgery, with our brass plate on the wall that read:

DR LIAM MEAGHER
DR LUCIA GANNON

GENERAL PRACTITIONERS

I returned to work after my maternity leave with a renewed sense of enthusiasm. On that first day, in my very own bright, spacious consulting room, I felt like a child in a toy shop. For the weeks prior to starting back, I had stolen a few hours each evening to set my room up exactly as I wanted it. My diplomas and certificates, which had been stored in a quiver-like case since my return from the UK, were finally displayed on the wall. My nameplate was attached to the door. My bookshelves contained reference books, guidelines and medical journals. An examination couch lay along one side of the room with an adjustable light attached to the wall above it. At the foot of the couch lay a trolley containing specula, dressings and urine bottles. In the corner was a sink, a paper-hand-towel dispenser and mirror. The long desk would eventually hold a computer and printer, but in those days it acted as a repository for the large number of paper files, reports and letters that were delivered daily. My final act of organisation before opening my door was to hang a Picasso print of a mother breastfeeding her baby on the wall behind my consulting chair. If a picture painted a thousand words, then that should save me a lot of talking. Slowly, I picked up where I had left off four months earlier, before Liam's birth. Gradually, the familiar patterns of consulting and examining were re-awakened until I felt as if I had never been away.

I do not recall who the first patient was in my very own consulting room, but I distinctly remember the last patient of the day, a woman in her forties who had been awaiting the return of the 'lady doctor', as she required a cervical smear test. She seemed nervous and unsure as to whether or not she should have come in. As a woman, I could relate to her reticence and anxiety. I had never forgotten how it had felt, years earlier, when I had presented myself for the same test to a doctor in the UK. I'd found myself in a room with a bare leather couch, no blanket, no blind, no curtain or screen, no light and no lock on the door. It had been a powerful lesson on how not to do something and I had vowed to be extra attentive to the privacy and dignity of patients when I had my own practice. In my own room, I was finally able to put that into practice. I had new couch roll for the couch, a blind for the window, a special adjustable light, a soft, brightly coloured blanket and a screen for additional privacy. I made full use of them all and when I was finished, I invited the woman to sit back next to my desk while I filled out the paperwork.

'Well, that was painless,' she said, smiling. 'I don't know why I put it off as long as I did.'

'We are all the same,' I replied. 'Everybody hates smear tests.'

I imagine that it was because she had faced her fear and conquered it that she felt she could explore the issue a bit more and asked me how many more years she would have to keep having the tests. I checked her age before I replied. 'About another twenty years or so, unless the guidelines change in the meantime.'

'That's a long time,' she said. I suppose you will see me out for smears then. I take it you intend to stay here and not move on?'

It was more of a statement than a question and it unsettled me. I was here and I did intend to stay, but twenty years was an awful long time. Was I really ready to say that I would stay in that village, in that surgery, seeing the same patients for twenty years? How could anyone ask me to commit to that? It was her certainty that disturbed me most, the hint of possessiveness in her voice that all of a sudden made me want to contradict her. 'Who knows,' I said, to hide my discomfiture. 'Who knows where any of us will be this time next year, never mind in twenty years' time.'

Early in our relationship, I had tried to explain my difficulty with decision-making and commitment to Liam. I liked to keep my options open. I didn't like to be too certain of my plans. I liked to leave room for the unexpected. Liam had worked as a bus conductor in Dublin during his summers as a student, so I used a bus analogy. 'It's as if I hate catching a particular bus. Once I get on that bus, then that's it, there is no chance of me catching another one. I have to wait until that one stops and by then, I might be somewhere that I don't want to be.'

He had looked at me as if I was speaking a foreign language. However, Liam was the eldest of three boys and his not having sisters meant that I could convince him that some of my strange ideas and behaviours were normal for women.

'But what about me?' he had asked. 'Why did you catch me?'

'You are not a bus,' I replied. 'You just happened to join me at the bus stop and I latched on to you as someone who might help me decide which one to take. You do know a lot about buses, after all.' Despite the fact that Liam and I had been in the same class in college for six years, a class of only fifty students, we had managed to avoid romantic entanglement until the end of our final year. Liam claimed that he had tried to attract my attention many times, but that I had given off a very definite air of disinterest. I accused him of not trying hard enough and that if it had not been for my creative manoeuvres, we would never have got together. This was one of many things we agreed to disagree on.

Once my last patient had left the room, I sat back in my chair, still feeling a little perturbed. Liam and I had definitely taken the same bus and had already gone a long way on our journey. In the field up the hill from the surgery, Liam had planted a mini-forest, a wind shield for the house we would eventually build on that site. Along with this forest, I was beginning to realise that we were planting ourselves firmly in this community. Since returning from the UK, seven years earlier, we had worked in GP practices all over the country, from Donegal to Wexford. We had worked in Thomastown, Co. Kilkenny, Kilkenny City and West Cork. I had been employed as a medical officer in a private hospital in Galway, a senior house officer in psychiatric hospitals in Kilkenny and West Cork and an area medical officer in the then South-Eastern Health Board. Liam and I had both done additional educational courses, completed extra examinations and studied for numerous diplomas.

On a particular lazy Sunday afternoon, I had helped Joseph count the number of houses he had lived in before he started school and finished with a total of nine. This wasn't because we liked moving around, or because we couldn't make up our minds about where to live: if we wanted to work in the same practice and treat public and private patients, one of us needed to be appointed to a General Medical Services (GMS) or medical card list. In 1991, the year that we returned to Ireland, the only way to get such a list was to take over from a GP who had retired or died, or to join an established GP as an assistant. Lists were in short supply and were awarded on the basis of an interview to eligible doctors, those who had already gained some GMS experience, usually by working in a small practice or as an assistant to another GP. Liam had first been appointed to a medical card list in 1994, in the small practice in Drimoleague, but Killenaule had the potential to accommodate us both.

A village in South Tipperary, on the Kilkenny–Cashel tourist trail, Killenaule is known best by some as the place where Sonia O'Sullivan won her first National Cross-Country Championship in 1987. Others knew it as a place they passed through on their way to visit the 'bonesetter', the late Jimmy Heffernan, a man rumoured to have performed miracle cures for all manner of ailments, who lived close by in the village of Drangan. I would come to know it and the surrounding townlands as they were depicted in the song 'The Hills of Killenaule', composed by Killenaule native the late Davy Cormack, along with Liam

O'Donnell, and sung by Louise Morrissey:

> 'Alone Slievenamon rules over all,
> Whose valleys Ballingarry enthral,
> It's nice in Fethard and Moyglass,
> And Coolmore of green-blue grass,
> But it's lovely 'round the hills of Killenaule.'

Killenaule was where we would see if it was all worth the effort. As I drove the short distance home after my first day in my own consulting room, in my own surgery, I allowed myself to consider that at the age of thirty-four, I might finally be embarking on real general practice and would not be catching any more buses.

CHAPTER THREE

THE HILL HOUSE

In the millennium year, two years after I had first sat in my own consulting room, two pillars stood sentry at the bottom of a driveway that curved upwards from the surgery to our new house, a driveway that skirted an old hawthorn tree that hung protectively above an ancient well. It wasn't an ancient well, of course – it had been drilled by the previous owner – but I liked to pretend that it was. I had read somewhere about the Celtic tradition of dipping rags in the water of ancient wells and hanging them on a hawthorn, or 'clootie tree', to dry. The rags symbolised ailments and as they rotted, the ailments would resolve and disappear. Apart from that, it is well known that a lone hawthorn tree serves as a meeting place for the fairies and that having such a tree on your property brings luck and prosperity. I liked to imagine that both the tree and the well were a sign that we had chosen a suitable place for our own healing endeavours. With its delicate white May flowers and deep-red autumn berries, this emblem of hope still blooms today among the laurel, elder, holly, beech and bramble.

Our newly built house had some features of the traditional farmhouses of the area and some others that our architect said had been influenced by the Scottish architect and designer Charles

Rennie Mackintosh. These included windows of varying shapes and sizes and a turret-style front porch with a conical roof. I had no prior knowledge of Mackintosh and had simply requested that we try to achieve a house whose structure was related to function: one of the few things I remembered from my histology lectures as a student was that the body was a perfect example of 'structure related to function' and, while a house is not the same as the body, I saw no reason why we could not apply the same principle. Despite this eclectic mix of styles, once completed, the house nestled into the hill as if it had always been there.

Being a peripatetic GP had a lot of advantages when it came to planning a house. I knew what I wanted: a conservatory, a pantry, a utility room, a study, a dresser for the kitchen, a cooker with a gas hob and electric oven; a large kitchen table with room for unexpected visitors and lots of bookshelves to accommodate our ever-increasing collection of books. As our lives and family expanded, so too did this collection, which, by then, contained an expanding children's section, a large adult fiction section, Liam's history and politics shelf, a new home and garden section and my 'how to' section, with its instructions on playing tennis, swimming, golfing, skiing, thinking, writing and even one that I usually filed with the spine hidden so that no one would see it, entitled *How to Read a Book*. In that pre-digital age, it was hard to imagine that a time would come when a whole library could be contained on a device the size of a single copy of F. Scott Fitzgerald's *The Great Gatsby*.

Before turning a sod in the field, Liam had visited our neighbours to show them the house plans and to reassure them that we would not overlook their gardens or obstruct their view. But there was one group that he did not think to consult: the brave and curious furry creatures, the rabbits, who had busied themselves underground for years and who came out of their homes to nibble at the bark and leaves of the tender young trees and shrubs. When satiated, they sat defiantly on the lawn or driveway, backs hunched, ears erect, signalling to us and to each other, 'This is our field and we will not give it up without a fight.' But whenever I complained about the damage they did, my children reminded me of the story of Fiver and Hazel in *Watership Down* and how they, with their small band of rabbits, had been forced to make a perilous journey to safety when the diggers attacked their field. We had brought the diggers into this field and it was up to us to make our peace with the rabbits and learn to co-exist, which we eventually did.

Just as we were becoming more familiar with our patients, piecing together the family connections and becoming accustomed to the local traditions and beliefs, so, too, were our patients getting to know us and our ways. With this familiarity came a sense of belonging and ease that I had not previously experienced in my work. It could, however, also have its downsides: familiarity led to advice, whether I asked for it or not.

'You would want to put a gate on those pillars,' a man called Mr Brennan said to me one day, as I was writing a note in his file at the end of our consultation. 'Something you could lock,' he went on. 'I was just having a look at them on my way in. There could be anybody cruising around here, you know. And with no gate, your house up there is an open invitation to robbers. You're making it very easy for them.'

Mr Brennan was a farmer who had good reason to be security conscious, as on a few occasions over the years he had had farm machinery stolen from his yard. I knew he was right, but I had not asked for his advice. Giving advice was what I got paid to do, even if, some days, it seemed as if I received more than I gave away. Some days, it felt as if the doctor–patient interaction was more of a trading relationship, as if, having received something, people liked to give something in return. But while they were actually asking for my advice, I was not asking for theirs and in those early days, I sometimes did not know how to say, 'thanks, but no thanks.'

In the course of a normal day I could receive advice on all manner of subjects, from housekeeping, gardening, to mothering and even fashion. 'I like your dress,' a lady said to me one day, as I was standing with my back to her washing my hands at the sink. 'But if you don't mind me saying, it's just a little bit long. It could do with a little stitch at the waist to tuck it up a bit.' As she spoke, she came towards me and before I knew it, she had grasped the back of my dress and folded a section of the waist between the thumb and forefinger of one hand. 'Just about that much,' she said. 'That would make all the difference.'

I thanked her while wriggling out of her grasp. She smiled back at me, obviously pleased with herself. I had no idea that that was what she was observing while I was busy washing my hands. Obviously, I wasn't the only one who noticed things. The dress, thereafter, hung unworn and unaltered in the wardrobe, before finally being put into a bag for the charity shop.

It was nice to be appreciated as a person, rather than simply a 'service provider'. It was nice that people cared enough to offer advice, but I wondered if there was something about me that encouraged people to help me, or correct me, or educate me on all manner of things. For as long as I could remember, I had consistently been told that I looked much younger than my years. This was both a blessing and a curse, depending on what I was trying to achieve. As a teenager, I was viewed with suspicion when I offered to babysit for one of the many families who came every summer to the holiday cottages in my childhood home of Tullycross, Renvyle, Co. Galway. I knew that behind the polite smiles of the parents lay the burning question, 'What age is she?' Sometimes, when I was feeling benevolent, I put them out of their misery early. I let others squirm and wriggle until they finally came straight out with it.

One evening when Liam and I were living in Thomastown, and I was in my late twenties, I answered the door to a patient. A man in jodhpurs and a riding jacket stood in the dim light of the porch. From the way he was holding his right arm across his chest, I deduced that he had probably fallen off his horse, possibly sustained a fracture and would need referral to the nearest emergency department. I ushered him into the hallway and told him to take a seat, saying I would be with him in a minute.

He did as I asked but gave me a puzzled look. 'Thank you,' he said. 'I'm sorry to call so late, but I was wondering is your daddy in? I need to see the doctor.'

I called my 'daddy' and left them to it. On that occasion it was definitely a blessing.

Thankfully, I was no longer mistaken for the doctor's daughter, but I thought that some people still had their doubts as to whether I was a fully qualified GP. As I walked from the surgery to the house one evening, I thought again about the advice that Mr Brennan had given me about the gates. I had wanted to tell him that we had our own reasons for not installing locked gates at the entrance to our house, but I hadn't been sure he would understand. We were country GPs and on our nights off, patients did not disturb us with trivial matters, but there was an unwritten understanding that if somebody collapsed, if a child had a seizure, if a teenager suffered an acute asthma attack, or if a mother suffered a post-partum haemorrhage, as well as calling an ambulance, they should contact us as soon as possible and we would do what we could, whether we were on call or not. We were lucky to have a rota with our colleagues in the neighbouring towns of Fethard and Ballingarry, which meant we were only on duty one night and one weekend in every four, but with the telephone switched to a neighbouring GP, the only way to contact us was by calling to the house and we did not want to create a situation where someone did not get necessary treatment because of a lock on a gate. The sentries were designed to stand alone.

If this decision did indeed save patients' lives, it could also have could have cost us our own child's life, if it were not for the kindness and vigilance of a stranger.

As I stood at the kitchen sink one evening, looking out absent-mindedly through the little narrow window, which had been strategically placed to allow a view of the front door, I saw a man I did not recognise about to ring the doorbell. He had a small child in his arms. I dried my hands and went to the door. The child he was carrying was my own two-year-old, Liam Jnr.

The man noted the look of horror and confusion on my face and obviously knew that he had come to the right house. 'It's OK,' he said quickly, as if afraid I would attack him for attempting to steal my son. 'He is fine. I just spotted him trying to cross the road.'

The main road was approximately eighty yards from our house, a big journey for a two-year-old. The man must have gone on to explain how he had come to pick Liam Jnr up, put him in his car and take him to our house, but I do not remember any of that. I do remember taking my child from him and realising that he was unharmed, feeling weak and frightened, relieved and confused, all at the same time. I am sure I must have thanked the man before he left, but it seemed that he was gone too soon and I was left trying to figure out how I could have let my two-year-old get as far as the main road without noticing.

As my heart rate settled, I gradually stopped the self-recriminations long enough to piece together the events of the evening. I had walked Joseph, then eight, across the road to the sports complex for hurling training. Liam Jnr had come with us. He had wanted to stay and play with the big boys, but I had too much to do, so I'd carried him home, Liam kicking and screaming in my arms. Always an easy personality, he had given up his struggle by the time I got home, so I'd put him down, closed the door behind me and had gone to answer the telephone, which had just started to ring. A short time later, I had answered the door to the man with the child. A short time that could have changed our lives for ever. To this day, I have no idea who the man was and even though I no longer shudder at the thought of what could have been, I still feel overwhelming gratitude for his actions.

My initial reaction was to insist we order gates and get someone to hang them the next day, but Liam, as usual, added perspective. He pointed out that if a child wanted to get down from our house to the hurling pitch, situated directly across the road from the surgery, there were lots of ways of avoiding locked gates. He also knew that we were in and out through those gates so often every day that they would never be closed, never mind locked. My rational brain knew he was right, but what kind of a mother was I if could not keep my children safe? I battled with these opposing views until much later, when I came to the realisation that my role was to educate Liam Jnr on the dangers of the world as I saw them. He would have to learn to navigate those dangers himself. Much and all as I wanted to, I could not make everything safe. As the months passed and it seemed as if my youngest child had no longer any desire to stray into dangerous territory, I conceded that his father was right.

'It's like that Buddhist quote you read out to me a couple of weeks ago,' Liam said. 'It was something about how having leather soles on your feet is easier than covering the whole world with leather.'

It was a recurring source of wonder and annoyance to me that Liam seemed to remember more of what I read than I did. I went in search of the quote by the Buddhist, Shantideva, and sure enough it was almost exactly as he had remembered it: 'With leather soles beneath my feet, it is as if the whole world has been covered.'

We could not cover the whole world with leather. Our children would have to develop their own soles.

CHAPTER FOUR

A GOOD TEACHER

Many years earlier, my own mother had tried to cover my
path with leather, but I had not taken the route that she
had prepared for me. My mother was a primary school
teacher who loved her job and thought that it was the perfect
fit for any woman who wanted to have children. The short days
and long holidays balanced the intensity of the concentration
required in the classroom and allowed time for home and family.
In her experience, it was unusual for mothers to work in other
professions.

The woman who I called my mother was actually my
stepmother. My biological mother had died suddenly at the age
of twenty-eight, when I was seven months old, leaving my father
with four children under the age of six. Years later, my sister
showed me a copy of my mother's death certificate. It stated
pulmonary embolism as the cause of death. She was admitted to
hospital one day with a cough and shortness of breath and never
came home.

A couple of years after this tragedy, my stepmother arrived in
Renvyle, my home place, by bicycle. She had come from a little
village called Errislannan, south of Clifden, to take up the post
of assistant teacher in Tully National School. As she had a very

long cycle from her home to Tully every day, the bicycle was quickly exchanged for a Honda 50, which subsequently had to be abandoned, following hints from some people that it might not be proper for a young female teacher to transport herself on a motorbike. This young, attractive, independent and strong-minded woman had no choice but to follow this advice and find digs. She had no trouble finding a family to take her in and we grew up with a sense of reverence for that same family, aware that they always held a special place in my mother's heart. This relocation was advantageous for my father and his four young children. A woman who, I was later told, could probably have had her choice of many a young man in the parish only had eyes for my father and he, having found love and happiness once, had no reason to believe he could not find it again. Despite warnings about the foolishness of taking on another woman's children, she married my father and became our mother.

At the age of twelve, I was sent to Coláiste Mhuire, Tourmakeady, a boarding school on the shores of Lough Mask in Co. Mayo. My older sister was already there. I would get my Leaving Certificate and then, all going to plan, would get a call to teacher training, preferably at Carysfort College in Dublin, where my mother had trained.

I liked the idea of becoming a teacher. I had seen my mother do it and figured I could do it, too. In those days, a call to training depended on having a reasonable Leaving Certificate, relatively good Irish, being able to sing reasonably well and play at least three tunes on a musical instrument. Tourmakeady was an Irish-speaking musical haven with a good academic record, so I embraced it all with enthusiasm. I loved being a team member, whether it was in a musical group, a choir or the debating team. I loved the recreation hall with its thick floor mats, balance beams and vaulting boxes, where I practised headstands and handstands for hours when it was too wet to go outside. I loved the challenge of taking a blank page, filling it with words, handing it over to my teachers and getting their reaction. Most of all, I loved the little music rooms that lined the corridor to the refectory. I would trade my Sunday afternoon bun for an additional half-hour of practice time on one of those pianos, each with its unique smell and feel and sound. In those rooms, I listened, with a mixture of awe and envy, to my much more accomplished classmates playing fiddles, tin whistles, accordions and guitars and tried to play as they did. In Tourmakeady, I learned that anything worth doing takes hard work and practice, but the joy of achievement makes it all worthwhile and despite the fact that I cried myself to sleep every night for the first year, I would not have given it up. By the time I left, fluent in Irish, with a lot more than the required three tunes and a large repertoire of songs, I was probably the most well-prepared potential teacher in the country.

As expected, I did get the call to training. It came in the form of a letter, delivered one day when my mother was in hospital in Galway, having her tenth baby, my youngest sister and the fourteenth member of our family. When she rang home, I gave her the news. I remember her saying, 'You will need a suit for the interview. Maybe come in with your father when he is next coming to visit and you can have a look around Galway.'

I had jumped the first hurdle, the academic achievement, but I still had to do an interview. I had not thought about a suit. I had never worn one in my life and I had rarely been shopping in Galway, so I had no idea where to look for one. My father was no help: he left me to fend for myself while he visited my mother in hospital. I presume his reasoning was that if I was going to go to college, I needed to start finding my way in the world. At seventeen, I could clean a house, babysit a family of six under-sixes, cook a dinner, quote Shakespeare, compare and contrast the writings of the various Brontë sisters, offer an opinion on apartheid in South Africa, but I had no idea what sort of a suit one would wear to an interview or how to go about getting one.

In Galway, I wandered in and out of shops with no idea what I was looking for and I was in bad form by the time I got back to the hospital, to find my father already there and my mother feeding the baby. My sister was a chubby little girl with a full head of black hair, unlike her siblings, who were all fair. My mother looked tired, so I took the baby from her, popped her on my shoulder and walked up and down between the hospital beds, patting her on her back, drinking in the new-baby smell, the softness of her skin and the perfection of her little face.

My mother noted the absence of shopping bags and asked why I had not bought anything. The fact was, I had not even tried anything on. I had no mental image of myself in a suit. I was short and slight with mousey-coloured shoulder-length hair. I was quite sure that nobody made suits for someone like me. But my mother had a plan. 'I wonder would your Aunty Geraldine have anything to fit you?' she mused out loud. 'I'm sure she would not mind you borrowing something.' Aunty Geraldine was my father's sister, who lived in Galway. She was only ten years older than me, but she might as well have been sixty. I was definitely not going to wear any of her suits.

My father suddenly looked up from the paper he had been reading since I came in. 'They have a place for you across the road,' he said, in a disinterested manner, as if he was just sharing a headline from the paper.

'Where?' asked my mother, before I could speak. 'In the university?'

'Yes,' replied my father, going back to his paper.

'Well they don't do teaching there,' my mother said. 'How do you know she got a place anyway?'

My father explained that he had gone to the Central Applications Office (CAO) in town and enquired as to whether I had received any offers of a university place. He said this as if it was something he did regularly. It always baffled me how my father knew things like this: how he could find his way around Dublin without a map, even though he hardly ever went there and how he would know that the CAO office was situated in Galway and that there might be a place for me in NUIG, when he had no experience of academia, as I would be the first in our family to apply to that system.

'So, what have I been offered?' I asked, trying to hide my annoyance that while I had been left shopping for a suit, he was checking out my future.

'Medicine,' he replied.

I remember that a whole host of new possibilities flashed before me. Up until that point, my future seemed pre-ordained and I had been happy with that, but with the news that I had been offered a different future came the weight of having to make a decision.

I became aware of my mother's voice. 'I didn't know you had medicine on your CAO form,' she said. 'I didn't think you would be interested in medicine.'

I explained that I wasn't really that interested. I had just put it down because others were putting it down and the teacher helping us with the forms said it would be no harm to tick it. In those days, getting into medicine was not quite as difficult as it is now. It still required hard work, but I enjoyed academic endeavour and simply aimed to do the best I could. Alongside medicine, I had also entered speech therapy and occupational therapy, although I had no idea what those jobs entailed.

My father asked if I thought I would like medicine as a career. My mother's tone, as she answered for me, suggested that this was a ridiculous question. 'Paddy,' she said, 'medicine is a long, hard course. It's twice as long as teacher training and it's very hard work. I see the doctors in here and they are dead on their feet. There is no way Lucia would be fit for that.'

I had stopped listening and must have looked pensive as my mother addressed me directly, drawing me back into the room. 'You're not seriously thinking of doing medicine?' she said, looking more than a little perturbed.

I'm not sure what I replied to her, but I was coming to a decision. If doing medicine meant I did not have to wear a suit that belonged to my Aunty Geraldine, then that was a good enough reason for me to do it.

The fact that that conversation took place in the postnatal ward of a maternity hospital did not strike me as significant until many years later. My mother had managed to give birth to ten children and raise fourteen, while holding down a full-time job as a teacher. I found out that I had a choice of medicine as a career while visiting her, after the birth of one of those children. It was as if the two options were being presented to me at once, so that I would be clear about my choices. Career, or children, or both? I knew teaching was compatible with motherhood, but there was a chance that medicine was not and this is what, I think, my mother was trying to convey to me. It was her attempt at keeping me safe.

Even at that young age, I could not imagine a life without children of my own. I had helped to raise all my younger siblings. With them I had felt, for the first time, the joy of unconditional love. Any affection I bestowed on them was returned a thousand-fold. At times when the loss of my birth mother threatened my equilibrium, the elusive loss that visited unbidden and had no name or focus, it was the kisses and caresses of these young siblings that kept my world safe and rich and fun. Their soft baby skin, their toddler giggles, their chubby arms around my neck when I came home from boarding school, their snuggling in beside me at night after I lifted them from their cot to soothe a bad dream or just let them know they were not alone, I knew I wanted this in my life. There was lots I did not know, but I was sure that at some point, I wanted to be a mother. Becoming a doctor might be something I could do until then.

I could not have imagined then that I would, in time, become both a doctor and a teacher, even if I was not the sort of teacher my mother had thought I would be. After a few years in practice in Killenaule, Liam returned from a meeting one day, asking if I would have any interest in applying for a post as a GP trainer on the South-East General Practice training scheme. This scheme had been established in 1991 by a group of committed and enthusiastic GPs with the support of the South-Eastern Health Board, as it was known then. The GP trainer role consisted of attending monthly workshops in Waterford and acting as a teacher and mentor to a GP registrar in our practice. (Registrars were qualified doctors who had completed at least one year's internship in hospital and had opted to join a structured GP training scheme.) My initial reaction to Liam's question was to reply that at times I just about knew what I was at myself, and could not imagine that I had the necessary skills or knowledge to teach others. Liam did not agree. By then we had employed Bernie, a practice nurse, but still had one free room that could be used for a GP registrar. Having another doctor in the practice would be good for us and for the patients, he thought. After all, we had designed our surgery with the intention of becoming a training practice if the opportunity arose. I suggested to Liam that perhaps he would be better at it than me. Part of me felt I had enough to do managing my own patients, helping Liam with practice administration and looking after three children, but part of me was also interested in trying something new. Liam said the decision was mine and he would support me either way, but he felt that I should be the one to do it. Liam knew that I enjoyed new challenges and thought that I would be suited to this one.

I reluctantly agreed to attend the interview for the position, but did not feel at all qualified for such a job. I was entering what was then an all-male domain, but felt encouraged by the fact that one of those men had suggested that I apply for the job. To my surprise, I was successful at interview and one Wednesday afternoon, I set out for my first trainer's workshop, in the training scheme offices on the campus of what was then known as Waterford Regional Hospital. I arrived early and met the other seven trainers on the scheme, all men. There was an air of semi-structured formality about the already well-established group, who had been meeting monthly for almost ten years by time I joined. I was welcomed with a mixture of open enthusiasm, genuine warmth and what I perceived as a hint of scepticism by some, but I was capable of imagining that.

In the company of these older men, I had to continuously remind myself that I was almost 36 years old and not a young, recently qualified, inexperienced doctor. In my first few workshops I oscillated between feeling confident and self-conscious, capable and deluded, young and old, experienced and inexperienced, open to all possibilities and challenges and wary of being found incapable. My inner critic whispered, 'imposter', and told me that I was just a token female, chosen only to narrow the gender gap. My rational brain told me that that was not true and that I was capable of learning new skills, just as all the other trainers had had to do. Part of me knew that I needed new challenges to stay interested in my career and that this was something I could learn to enjoy. So, despite my ruminations and self-doubt, I had to admit that I also felt alert, enthusiastic and interested. Little by little, my self-consciousness faded, my doubts subsided and my inner critic quietened, as I realised that I had not simply been chosen as a token female, but that the group was interested in my insights and ideas and that I could add value.

In addition to the trainers in the workshop, there were three programme directors, who oversaw the organisation of the training scheme for the Health Board. I learned later that female registrars referred to this team as 'the Vatican', as they were also an all-male group, and to the trainers as 'the bishops'. As I became more confident and interested, I felt drawn towards the Vatican. One day, I heard that they might be looking for someone new to join them, so I paid them a visit to find out more. While I enjoyed one-to-one teaching in the practice, I was more interested in facilitating small-group teaching and that was what the programme directors did. Before long, I had joined the cardinals in the Vatican. My new job as assistant programme director meant that I could no longer be a GP trainer and, after some discussion, Liam was persuaded to apply for the vacancy that I'd left and became a bishop. In this way, our country practice joined a network of interesting and supportive GP colleagues, who were committed not only to providing good-quality care for patients, but also to ensuring that there would be a stream of highly skilled GPs to come in their wake.

When I told my mother that I had taken on the additional role of teacher, she could not resist a satisfied 'I told you so.'

SAFETY-NETTING

The last of the evening sun was disappearing behind the beech hedge. A pile of unread post and lab results lay in a defiant pile to my left.

'See you tomorrow,' Bridget called as she left, pulling the door behind her with a bang.

I pushed the pile of papers further along the desk, slipped the CD, *Mavis Beacon Teaches Typing,* into the slot in the computer and waited for it to open on the screen. The computer, a new addition to our team, was as big and bulky as an old-fashioned television. It sat on the desk that extended almost the length of my room. I loved my long, spacious desk. It meant that paperwork could get pushed along to the furthest corner and stay there indefinitely, without disturbing my sense of order.

Mavis prompted me to begin my next lesson. Typing was my latest project. According to Liam, I have an addiction to 'projects', but as long as it just involves me, he doesn't mind. I had, at one time, tried to convince the whole family to practice Stephen Covey's *The 7 Habits of Highly Effective Families,* but that had ended prematurely, with me tossing the book into a charity shop bag in frustration, much to the family's relief. From then on, I stuck to setting challenges only for myself and typing was one of those. There was a beginning, middle and end; I started with no words on the page and finished with a readable document. I began at four words per minute but the more I practised, the faster I got. I had a definite goal, to type as fast as Bridget, keeping my eyes on the screen as she did, and to produce the rapid, rhythmic, soothing sound that she did, not my own stop-start sound, which assaulted rather than soothed my senses.

I was making slow but measurable progress, unlike in my consultations, where the more patients I saw and the more problems I was presented with, the deeper I felt I sank into the swirling ocean of unpredictability, uncertainty and confusion. Tasks were never completed, patients probably never satisfied. The more I came to know, the more I knew I did not know. Life was a constantly expanding to-do list, where very little ever got ticked off. And I liked ticking things off. I sometimes put things on my list after I had them completed just so that I could give myself the reward of ticking them off a minute later; little victories that fooled me into thinking I was in control.

The sound of someone entering through the front door disturbed my concentration. I stopped typing, hoping it was Bridget, back for some forgotten item. It wasn't. Bridget had forgotten something alright; she had forgotten to lock the door.

'Hello,' I heard from the waiting room.

I froze. I recognised that voice. It was far too familiar. I wanted to hide, but the door to my room was open and the owner of the voice was making her way towards me. It was too late. 'Hello,' I said back, getting out of my seat, sticking my head out of the door. She wasn't going to get into my room, I thought. I would not be held prisoner. I would keep advancing and get her out of the front door in sixty seconds flat and lock it behind her. What could she possibly want at six o'clock in the evening? I managed a smile. 'Well, is it yourself?' I said. 'Did you come to collect something? I'm just about to lock up and go home.'

She kept advancing towards me. In defence, I blocked the door to the consulting room, my arms extending outwards, holding the door frame on either side as I leaned out towards her, aware that despite my smile, my body language was definitely saying, 'Don't come any closer.'

'Oh, I'm so glad to catch you before you went home, Doctor,' she said in a downbeat, monotonous voice, out of keeping with her demeanour of forced cheer. She was, by then, up beside me, right in my space, so that I had no choice but to lower my arms and step back into the room. She shuffled past me, her head lowered, and sat down heavily on the chair beside my desk. No apology for the time of day, or the lack of an appointment. No acknowledgement that she might be interrupting me in the middle of something important.

What did you expect? I said to myself. Nothing is ever more important to her than herself and her imaginary problems.

I stood for a minute at the door, reluctant to follow her. If I sat down in my chair, she would have me exactly where she wanted me: in my consulting seat, giving her my undivided attention. That was the last thing I wanted, a consultation with someone who had not even bothered to book an appointment and who looked the picture of health, but I was no match for her. Perhaps the extent of her self-absorption prevented her from reading my body language or, having read it, she chose to ignore it. It didn't much matter. It appeared to be irrelevant.

'I'm so glad I got you, Doctor,' she went on. 'I'm not well at all. It nearly killed me to walk over. Not a bit well in myself.'

I sighed and sat down, determined to make this as short as possible. If only Bridget had locked the door, I thought. Outside, the sun had disappeared, the chirping of the birds had been replaced by the sound of homebound traffic. My typing lesson was half-finished on the computer, my dinner would be getting cold. The chemist was closed, in the unlikely event that she did need medication. I was trapped. I registered that she was talking, that someone looking on might even think that I was listening. I could also tell that there was nothing seriously wrong with her. Nothing that could not have waited until morning. Finally, I realised that it was my own fault. I should have gone home while I had the chance. I tuned in, in time to hear, 'So, you'll just have to give me something, Doctor. I can't go on like this.'

I looked into her smiling, expectant face, as familiar to me as that of one of my own children and wondered how many times I had heard her utter those same words.

If, on one of her many visits to the surgery, Bridget had a chance to intercept her at the reception desk, she would say, 'Doctor Gannon is fully booked today,' with an air of finality.

'Oh, I don't mind who I see,' would come the reply. 'I'll take the new, young doctor, if they have a free slot.' Looking around the waiting room, she would squeeze herself into the most densely occupied area, where she would relay her symptoms to anyone within earshot, before recounting those same symptoms, plus a few extras that she'd just thought of, all over again to the doctor. I tried to keep her away from the 'new, young doctor', if at all possible. Patients like this lady were challenging enough for a relatively experienced doctor, but they were certainly not suitable to be handed over to the young, soft-spoken, sensitive and conscientious registrar who was currently with us. A girl who, I had already decided, needed saving from herself, if she was to survive in general practice. I had been a bit like her in the early days: promising too much and not being able to deliver, harbouring aspirations of curing people like this lady, being the person to find the one thing wrong that all the other doctors had missed, sending the patient happily on their way, forever grateful, forever in my debt, their suffering ended. Another one ticked off the illness list.

My mother had a saying that she repeated frequently throughout our childhood. 'God help your innocent head.' I would smile smugly at whatever sibling she was addressing. It was never me. As a child, I kept my musings to myself, my questioning of the world well below the radar. I would not offer any hostages to fortune. I had a reputation as Little Miss Sensible and I found that in order to protect this reputation, it was best to say very little. I had, however, repeated my mother's phrase to myself many times as an adult.

Even though at that point I had been a GP for over ten years, I was still struggling with many of the more complex aspects of general practice, those that only really arise when treating the same patients over a sustained period of time, as I was doing in Killenaule. It was taking me many lessons to realise that some things were incurable; that there was a difference between caring for the person and curing the disease; that many people can have illness without an identifiable disease; that worrying about disease can be an illness in itself and that my job was to try and alleviate the suffering caused by this, without causing harm; that the care I provided had to be unconditional – it could not depend on someone getting better or responding to treatment. Unlike hospital specialists I could not say, 'Well, that's it. I've had a look inside, reviewed the test results, taken out the offending tumour and everything is tip-top. Off you go. No need to see me again.'

My most frequently repeated phrase was probably, 'Everything seems OK, but be sure and come back and see me if you are not well, or if anything changes.' It's called 'safety-netting'. Sharing the uncertainty. As a GP, I needed to let people know that I might be right, but on the other hand, I might be wrong. This is the right/wrong tightrope that I, and other GPs, walk in many consultations. No wonder some patients are more confused leaving than they were coming in.

On that evening, I tried my best to remain cheerful and caring, but my battery was low and I had used up my store of creative solutions for that day. I tried to remind myself that despite her frequent attendances and insatiable desire for medical attention, this lady was generally pleasant and appreciative. But she was taking up far too many consultations. This was probably the hundredth time I had seen her that year and it was only September. A pain in her stomach, a pain in her head, a tingling in her leg, a dizzy feeling, a fluttering in her heart, a ringing in her ear, a shadow in her eye, no appetite, tired all the time, not sleeping, sleeping too much, a sick feeling, an all-over itch, pins and needles in her fingers. The list was endless.

'Do you ever think that you might be a little depressed?' I asked her on more than one occasion.

'No, Doctor. Why would you think that?'

'I'm only asking,' I replied. 'But maybe depressed is the wrong word. Maybe a little over-anxious about your health?'

'Oh, no, Doctor. Once you tell me it's nothing to worry about, then I don't worry. I'm not anxious at all.' She smiled happily. She could see what I was trying to do. She knew that I was angling to share the burden with a psychiatrist or a counsellor. This was an avenue that she had no intention of entering and deftly blocked.

I was pretty sure there was nothing serious wrong, but eventually, someday, something would go wrong and I didn't want a repeat of Spike Milligan's infamous epitaph, '*Dúirt mé leat go raibh mé breoite*' ('I told you I was ill'), inscribed on this lady's gravestone, a permanent reminder of my incompetence. On the other hand, I couldn't examine her fully every time I saw her, and in any case, no amount of examination provided reassurance. No amount of reassurance stopped her coming back within the week, shuffling in, her latest symptoms laid out before me like a cat presenting a gift to its owners. Her brain was continuously scanning for bodily discomforts, and her neural pathways appeared to be on a continuous loop: symptom, disease, doctor, symptom, disease, doctor. I tried to put myself in her shoes, to imagine what it must be like to live as she did, always one symptom away from a terrible disease. Perhaps I would be the same, if I didn't have a medical degree.

'There is nothing wrong with you,' I was tempted to say on more than one occasion, but that would be tempting fate. 'I can't find anything wrong with you,' was more my style, even though I knew this was frequently misinterpreted as a failing on my part. Nevertheless, I had to be true to myself. The scientist in me would not allow me equate 'no evidence of disease' with 'evidence of no disease', no matter how many times this lady attended. I had consulted the medical literature and read the numerous guidelines on managing the frequent attender. Just as I often explained to patients who enquired about cough bottles or treatments for a colicky baby that the reason there were so many remedies for these conditions is that none of them worked, likewise, the reason there were so many guidelines written for patients like this lady was that they rarely worked. In reality, frequent attenders were as diverse as snowflakes. No two were the same. I would have to compile my own guidelines for this lady, I thought, as we both sat there. Perhaps she could be another of my projects, I mused. If I found a way to deal with her, I could write it up.

I stopped myself. I was going down a familiar route, a blind alley that would lead nowhere. You can't change other people's behaviour, I reminded myself. You can only change your response. I became aware, once more, that she was speaking. 'Just a minute,'

I interrupted her. 'I need to get your file.' As she did not have an appointment, her name was not on my list.

I left her sitting in my room and went into the reception area. I stood in front of the paper files in the filing cabinet behind the reception area. Rows and rows of them, fat ones, thin ones, all in brown cardboard covers, some with spines broken, the contents sticking out, making it difficult for me to open the cabinet door. As I moved my fingers from right to left, I suddenly realised I didn't know what file I was looking for. I couldn't remember her name. A woman who had been attending me twice weekly for almost four years and I couldn't, without a prompt, remember her name. I pulled out a few fat files, knowing hers would be one of these and hoping for inspiration, but this only made it worse. I sat on the floor behind the reception desk, thinking, going through the alphabet in my head, but her name refused to come to me. Eventually, I went back to my room, opened the list of registered patients on the computer and scanned the list, hoping for a clue, but still, my mind remained blank. I gave up trying, in the hope that it would suddenly pop into my head and conducted the rest of the consultation in a state of distraction. I don't think she noticed, such was the extent of her self-absorption and when eventually I sent her on her way, I was more worried about myself and my memory loss than I was about her.

That evening, at dinner, it suddenly came to me. 'Kitty O'Dwyer,' I exclaimed. 'Thank God. Kitty O'Dwyer. I thought I was going crazy, but that's it, Kitty O'Dwyer. How could I not have remembered her name?' No one took any notice of my outburst. I was obviously pleased with myself about something. When I didn't say any more, they resumed their eating and conversation and I finished my meal, relieved and smiling to myself.

One day, some months later, I was shopping in the local supermarket. I was moving purposefully around the aisles, keeping myself to myself, when I heard a loud and animated conversation coming from somewhere near the deli counter. I stayed where I was, eavesdropping, examining the cereal, like an undercover detective. The shop could be a useful source of additional information on patients: the man who claimed to have quit smoking six months earlier might be stuffing his newly bought pack of Silk Cut into his pocket; the woman who 'never touches a drop' could be furtively slipping a baby Powers into her shopping bag. The whiskey could be for anyone: it's the manner in which it would be deftly and swiftly hidden from sight that was the giveaway.

On that particular day, the voice I heard was telling a funny story, something about a dog called Ben, who somebody thought was a human because of the name, and the confusion that arose as a result. Loud guffaws of laughter interrupted the flow of the narrative, contagious laughter that caused other shoppers to snigger and peer around the aisles to see who was responsible for it. I did not need to look. I knew it was Kitty. Kitty, who I had never heard laugh, who had never told me a funny story, who, I would have thought, had never even heard a funny story. Kitty, who spent her days worrying about her health and whose nights were filled with sleeplessness and anxiety. This same Kitty was holding forth with such gusto and zeal and obvious enjoyment of her story that she was barely recognisable.

Well, I thought to myself. There is joy in her life. It's just not shared with me. I put my box of Weetabix into my basket and stepped around the corner, revealing myself. 'Well, ladies,' I said. 'You can't beat a good laugh. Better than any medicine.'

Kitty seemed surprised to see me. 'Oh, hello, Doctor,' she said, but I could swear I saw her demeanour change, her shoulders droop and her brain once again register her numerous discomforts. I left before I stole her joy.

After that, I didn't worry so much about Kitty. Her laughter reassured me that she was at ease in her world. What she presented to me in each short consultation was a little tip of the tip of her iceberg. Her life was as full and engaging and rewarding as any other. I could never find a cure because there was no ailment. At least not yet. I was simply a player in her drama, a bit-player who added a bit of colour, a bit of variety.

I slowly and steadily changed my response to Kitty. The strategy I evolved for dealing with this lady was not in any book. I was not even aware that it *was* a strategy. In my head I just gave up, resigned myself to my fate, but what I actually did was become an absent doctor. I sat in my chair, I adopted a listening pose, I nodded and mumbled 'yes' and 'OK' at appropriate intervals. I leaned forward, feigning interest, or sat back pensively as the situation demanded. I examined sometimes, if I thought it was necessary, or other times when I could not think of anything else to do, but all the while, I was not present. Consultations became easier, if not exactly satisfactory, because I struggled with the idea that I might have lowered my standards, that I was not trying hard enough.

I was no longer trying to change her behaviour, no longer expecting to find a solution to her problems. What I was doing was learning acceptance, that what I wished for others was not necessarily what they wished for themselves and if they were going to worry unnecessarily about their health, there were times when I just had to let them do it. At least that prevented me from feeling drained, disappointed or frustrated. The strategy I developed for dealing with Kitty was necessary if I was to continue to see her. In time, I learned to accept that my main role with someone like her was to protect against over-diagnosis, over-investigation and over-treatment, while making sure I did not miss significant illness.

In hindsight, I see that the task of helping her to live with her imperfect health and reassuring her, without telling untruths or withholding information, was as intricate, delicate and important a function as alleviating symptoms or curing disease. I learned a lot from Kitty, even if she was totally oblivious to the contribution she made to my education.

Kitty would probably still be attending today, had she not left the area a few years ago to live with her sister in the Midlands.

'It was great having you here, Doctor,' she said, the last time I saw her, 'but you know, it was a bit far for me to walk to the surgery from my house. My sister's house is just around the corner from her doctor.'

'And have you checked if they will take you on?' I asked, realising that despite the frustration she engendered in me at times, I was actually fond of her and hoped she would find a doctor whom she could relate to. 'If they will, be sure and let me know, so that I can arrange to send on your file.'

'I'm sure they will,' she replied, full of confidence. 'There are a few of them in it. I'll surely get one of them to see me. But don't worry about the file. They will hardly need that. Sure, there couldn't be much in it. You never found anything wrong with me.'

No one ever looked for her file.

CHAPTER SIX

THE GIFT OF FRIENDSHIP

It was Jim's third consultation in two weeks. He was not a habitual attender, but on checking his file, I noticed that his consultation rate had increased considerably in the past few months. I had listened, examined, explained and reassured, but I was getting nowhere. I had checked his urine and arranged blood tests, just to be sure I was not missing anything, but everything was normal. I knew there was something bothering him and was pretty sure I knew what it was, but I couldn't find a way to broach the subject.

I knew that it was not me who was missing something. Three months earlier, Jim's best friend, Sean, had died. Sean, in his early sixties at the time of his death, was almost twenty years younger than Jim. He had been diagnosed with cancer and in the space of six months had gone from a healthy, active man to a terminally ill patient. At first, he lost his appetite and began to lose weight. Then he complained of pain in his abdomen and his skin developed a slight yellow tinge. On a wet October evening, he was admitted to hospital and he never came home.

When he came to see me, complaining of a pain in his right leg that kept him awake at night, Jim appeared to be coping well with his friend's illness. Having lost both his wife and his brother in the previous two years, Jim was no stranger to grief. Over those two years, he had oscillated between anger, denial, sadness and acceptance. He had grieved in his own way, but he had grieved and there was nothing abnormal about it. It was not protracted or curtailed. It just was. Sean's death was different. Jim appeared more sanguine, as if acceptance had come early without the other intervening stages. Or perhaps he was just not capable of further grieving.

'We were great friends,' Jim had said to me more than once since Sean's death, a statement that contained gratitude, sorrow and a hint of bewilderment. Jim would never have expected that Sean would be the first to die. Sean was the younger, stronger, healthier of the two, but in their relationship, they were equals. They simply enjoyed each other's company. Living in an isolated part of the country they were two of a group of men who would go to the local pub two or three times a week, have a couple of pints and go home. With the introduction of the new drink-driving laws and the risk of being over the legal driving limit, that practice had to stop, so, Sean would sometimes stop by Jim's house in the evening for a cup of tea and a chat and gradually these visits took the place of the pub. There was always something to discuss. Who was buying land from whom? How would Tipperary do in the hurling? How soon would the pub close due to lack of customers? How were their children and grandchildren getting on and who would win the next election? I imagined that there were very few topics that had not been discussed in that little kitchen. I also imagined that Jim had a huge void in his life where Sean had been, a void that could not be filled by family or other friends. I wondered how he passed his evenings and if he sometimes anticipated Sean's step in the hall or his loud knock on the sitting room door, announcing his arrival.

I suspected that Jim's physical pain had its roots in unacknowledged grief. Perhaps his head was telling him that it was good that Sean did not suffer, but his heart had lost another life support. His world had changed. Another connection had come undone and he had no blueprint for dealing with it.

Now I turned to Jim and decided to be straight about what I thought was the cause of his health worries. 'Jim, are you missing Sean?' I asked.

He gave me a startled look, as if I had just hit him across the face, his eyes wide, his mouth a thin line, lips pressed tightly together, with just a hint of trembling. After what seemed like a long time, he spoke. 'I feel so guilty,' he said. 'I feel so angry and guilty and … ' He stopped and looked down at his lap, unable to go on.

'And sad?' I suggested gently.

He nodded. I felt that his grieving had just begun.

Jim's reluctance to grieve had made me wonder if there was a special type of grief that one experiences for a friend. Was it an invisible, lonelier feeling that did not attract the same level of support or understanding as that for a family member? I wondered if grieving for a friend was perceived as self-indulgent, an unnecessary burden on the bereaved family, which needed to be kept from view, buried deep out of sight. Who would we turn to, when the one we have always turned to is gone? Are we even aware of the importance of friends in our lives, until they are taken away, I wondered.

I had lots of practice at saying goodbye to friends. I had moved lots of times to new places and started all over again where nobody knew anything about me. I knew the emotional labour involved in making new friends and the loneliness of finding myself friendless. In 1994, two years before arriving in Killenaule, Liam and I had moved from Kilkenny, where we had been working for over two years, to the village of Drimoleague, in West Cork. It was the first step on the GMS list ladder and the most logical next step for us, if we were ever to establish our own practice. We left behind a recently established network of friends, work colleagues and neighbours, as well as playmates for Joseph, who, at two, was already competing for a place on the soccer team of ten-year-old boys who congregated on the common green in the housing estate where we lived. We left behind the bright, modern and comfortable house that we had been renting and moved to another rented premises, a dark, refurbished farmhouse on the side of a country road, with Joseph and his three-month-old sister, Ailshe.

For the first six weeks, Liam was on call seven days a week, twenty-four hours a day. Effectively, this meant that the whole family was confined to base, as there were not many places I could go with a baby and a two-year-old. Every day, Liam donned his work clothes and headed to the surgery, while I continued the endless round of feeding, changing, tidying, shopping and cooking that come with a toddler and a newborn. In the evenings, I walked up and down and up and down the long, low-ceilinged sitting room, with its small, deep windows and its fireplace at either end, because it used to be two rooms, rocking my baby in my arms, while singing 'Nellie the Elephant', over and over, the only rhythm that soothed her. Once she settled, I would sit with her in the over-sized lime-green armchair, with Joseph on my other side, while I read and re-read the adventures of Harriet the horse, Bert the bear and Dizzy the frog, from a children's book entitled *Tell Me a Story* bought on one of my few trips out to Skibbereen. During that first rain-soaked summer of 1994, when there were only the four of us, with no friends, no family and no work colleagues, my world became as grey as the omnipresent clouds, my only view the dense mist that seemed to hang permanently just a few feet from our kitchen window. I grew irritable, snappy and tired, my mood flat, my usually clear, optimistic and practical thinking caught in an unfamiliar negative loop. I knew from my medical training that I fitted some of the criteria for the development of postnatal depression: social isolation, no family support, career and financial uncertainty and a colicky baby. However, knowing these things did not mean that I felt their effects less intensely and rationalising my feelings did not make them go away. I knew I needed something to halt the downward spiral of negativity, but I did not know what that was.

One such gloomy day, I walked the short distance from our house to the village, one hand pushing Ailshe in her buggy, the other holding Joseph by the hand. As I descended the hill, I noticed two women standing at the entrance to a house on the opposite side of the road, chatting and laughing together. Their obvious ease in each other's company heightened my sense of loneliness. I didn't envy them: I just felt sad for myself as I was reminded of what I was missing.

As we came closer, the women stopped talking and one of them called out a friendly hello. 'Hello,' I called back, unsure what to say next, my social skills rusty, my motivation for making new acquaintances low. So, I simply smiled and kept going, as if I had an important errand to complete. The walk to the village was short, however, and in no time at all I was walking back up the same hill, reluctantly heading for home. The women were still there and as I was on the same side of the road as them, I knew I would have to engage. I braced myself.

One of the women stepped forward. She looked to be in her early forties, about ten years older than myself, with black shiny hair, cut stylishly short, dark brown eyes and almond-coloured skin. She looked alive and happy and full of enthusiasm, a painful contrast to what I was feeling. 'You are the doctor's wife,' she said.

It wasn't a question. It was more of a statement that did not require a response, as if she knew instinctively that I was not really up to introducing myself or to making small talk. 'And these are your two little ones.' She peered into the buggy where Ailshe, by then a thriving six-month-old, was sleeping, before turning to Joseph. 'And you,' she said. 'What's your name?'

Joseph moved away and hid behind my legs. She straightened up and addressed me. 'I'm Susan,' she said, 'and this is Margaret and we were just going to go in to have a cup of tea. Would you like to come in with us?'

It was the first invitation to connect that I had received since arriving in Drimoleague, almost three months earlier and I welcomed it as one would a drink of cool water on a hot and thirsty day. I followed the women in past two great big Labradors, stretched out sleepily on either side of the front door. I pushed the sleeping Ailshe into the hall, where she was promptly woken by the loud chirping of the two birds that hung in a cage overhead. I lifted her out of her buggy, only to have her taken from me instantly by a girl of about twelve, with hazel-green eyes and the same dark hair and skin as her mother.

'Look how blue her eyes are, Mam,' the girl said to her mother, while bouncing the smiling baby on her hip. The action reminded me of a much younger me, who would have done the same thing, in a similar manner, at her age. A me who had found joy in babies and toddlers, without the weight of responsibility that I felt now. I gladly left Ailshe in her capable hands.

Just then, two young girls, aged possibly six and eight, appeared from the kitchen and promptly moved Joseph out of the path of a fully uniformed Power Ranger, complete with sword, making a dash for the garden. 'Let's go after James,' one of them said, but Joseph was already in hot pursuit. I felt a weight lifting from my shoulders. This was a scene I was familiar with, a busy, bustling, bright and happy house where children entertained each other and adults had time for a cup of tea. I had not experienced this since I left my own home in Renvyle.

'Are they all yours?' I asked Susan, even though I already knew the answer. There was no mistaking their striking good looks.

'Indeed they are,' she said, 'all nine of them. And you're welcome to borrow any of them any time you want.' She busied herself plugging in the kettle and clearing a place on the counter, where she put three cups. Margaret moved two chairs closer to the table and indicated where I should sit down. 'Maura,' Susan called to an older girl, who appeared to be in the process of folding laundry in a back kitchen. 'Would you mind keeping an eye to the yard, the little fellah is gone off out there with the young ones.'

Maura smiled at me and went willingly to check.

I sat at the table and let my gaze wander out through the window to the front yard. It was the first time in three months that I did not have a child attached to some part of me. I looked up towards the sky and noticed that the clouds had parted and a small ray of sunshine had broken through. For the first time in a long time, everything did not seem so grey.

While I lived in West Cork, I did go back to work, but not as a general practitioner, instead going back to hospital, working as a psychiatric senior house officer in Skibbereen, but I was not happy there. I missed general practice: the pregnant women anticipating their new arrivals, the children with their talk of school and Santa and the older people with their practical wisdom. I felt that I was losing the skills I had worked so hard to attain. Killenaule was also closer to both our families than West Cork and later that year, Joseph would be starting school. So, despite the physical and emotional work of uprooting our family once again, we decided that it was the best decision for us. However, the connection we made with Susan and her family and, through her, with others in the community, brightened all our days and enriched our lives for ever.

In Killenaule, I once again faced the challenge of making new friends. I had been lucky to meet Judith while I was still relatively new to the village. She was not a patient at our practice, so that made the relationship easier. Making friends as a country GP is not straightforward. I cannot trade in gossip and I cannot talk about my work. I steer clear of medical topics, having found myself too many times in the middle of a conversation, only to realise that it has turned imperceptibly into a medical consultation and that I am working harder than I would in the surgery. In the early days of my practice, I felt I had to protect my boundaries. I needed to be able to answer my phone when I was not on duty and know that it was not going to be a request for medical advice. I avoided social settings where I did not feel I could mingle freely, be myself, or let my guard down. I did not want to disclose anything about anyone that could be interpreted as a breach of confidentiality – and I was not naturally extroverted. Rural practice is a tightrope. On the one hand, there is a need for connection and a sense of belonging, on the other a need to be objective, discreet, impartial and professional both inside and outside the surgery.

One day, as I was walking through the waiting room, my mind already on the next task, I noticed a woman, with a child of about ten, sitting waiting for an appointment with Liam. I recognised the woman. She had recently moved to the area from Waterford and was working as a nurse in the emergency department of the hospital in Clonmel. I nodded at them both and carried on with my day. Later, Liam came home with a jar of blackberry jam that the woman and her daughter had given to him as a gift for me. I was surprised and pleased and made a mental note to thank her when I next saw her.

The following day at lunch, I took the jam from the pantry, intending to have some. I was just about to open it, when I stopped. This wasn't just a simple jar of homemade jam, it was a work of art. The lid was covered with fabric in a mixture of autumn colours, held in place by an elastic band covered with a deep-green ribbon, tied in a perfect bow. A white label was stuck on the jar with the words, BLACKBERRY JAM. SEPT. 2004, written in an ornate deep green that matched the ribbon. At that moment, I was back in Mrs O'Toole's shop in Tullycross, looking longingly at the jars of homemade blackberry and raspberry jam lined up along a counter that was almost as high as my head. Mrs O' Toole's jam had never been as well presented as this.

I put the jar down and savoured its perfection. Something in that gift made me more than a little curious about the person who had given it. Something in that gift suggested a thoughtful, creative and mindful person, who had generously shared something of herself with me. Sitting at the table, I was reminded of the times when I was new to an area, without a sense of belonging and I resolved not to ignore a potential bid for connection, to reach out and take a risk, regardless of the obstacles.

A couple of years later, Dolores, the woman who had given me the jam, and I were sitting in her kitchen with her twin sister Kitty, who was visiting for a few days.

'So tell me,' Kitty said, sitting back at the table, her cup poised in her hand, 'how does it work when your friends need medical advice? Do you make them come to the surgery, or could they just ask you over for a cup of tea?'

Dolores shot her a look that said, that is none of your business. 'If you're hinting that you want medical advice,' Dolores said, 'then I have to tell you that you can expect to be charged and I will need a commission for supplying the venue.'

'No, I don't want any advice,' Kitty replied in a typically sisterly tone. 'I'm just interested to know what Lucia would do if a friend rang her up when she was not on duty and asked her to have a look at her child? I know *you* wouldn't do it, Dolores,' she said, emphasising the 'you', while looking directly at Dolores, 'but some people might think it was OK.'

Kitty was genuinely interested in how I navigated this tricky area and her questions were valid. I tried to explain that asking me to look at a sick child was not the same as asking me what was ailing a friend's aloe vera plant; that responding to a medical request involves a whole shift of mental energy. As a doctor, I work in the full knowledge that any sick child can suddenly become sicker. A child who is sitting up, chatting, in an emergency department can need resuscitation by the time they get to the ward. Every medical encounter deserves a history, an examination and a management plan and the full attention of the doctor involved. Once a mother decides her child needs a medical opinion, it elevates the implied level of concern. I need to respect my friends' abilities to make their own decisions as to when to get medical advice and not make them feel they need my opinion every time. I finished by saying that mothers need to be allowed to be mothers, friends friends, and doctor's advice confined to the surgery.

'Jeepers,' Kitty replied, 'it's a very complicated business. How did you two ever become friends with all those things to consider?'

Dolores suggested that it helped that we were both medical and understood the importance of confidentiality and the need to be really off duty when not working.

I thought about that and while that was probably true, I felt it was secondary. 'It was a jar of blackberry jam,' I said.

'I didn't know my jam was that good,' Dolores replied, raising her eyebrows and looking at me in surprise.

'Of course your jam is good,' I replied, having tasted more than one variety over the years. 'And so are your chutneys and crab apple jelly, but it is one particular jar I am talking about. One that you probably do not even remember giving to me.'

Nowadays, I count myself blessed with the many friends I have made. All friendships have boundaries, not just doctors', and all require commitment. As a GP, I meet a lot of people every day, so I am never at a loss for social interaction, but time with friends, whether it is walking, eating, meeting in our monthly book club, or simply talking on the phone, is something I cherish all the more because I know what it is like not to have it.

CHAPTER SEVEN

LEARNING A NEW LANGUAGE

I realised, shortly after coming to Killenaule, that if I wanted to be fully integrated into the community, I needed to expand my interests, increase my knowledge and learn a whole new language: that of the Gaelic Athletic Association, or GAA. This was not in any way related to medicine, but was very important for connection. 'A great match at the weekend', was as frequent a statement as, 'fair cold weather we are having', but while I knew something about the weather, I was often at a loss to know what match the person was talking about. The statement could be referring to Killenaule or Tipperary, to any age group from under-six to minor, under-21 or senior level. It could be a league, a championship or a challenge match. It could be hurling or football. It could be A or B division. My head could not make sense of the dizzying number of possibilities for any one 'match'. I usually kicked for touch and nodded in agreement, acceding to the superior knowledge of the speaker, not wishing to reveal the extent of my own ignorance.

In the surgery, boys and girls of all ages proudly wore their club or county colours. Red and yellow for Killenaule, or the 'Robins' as they are known, blue and gold for Tipperary. Every year, Santa would bring hurleys, sliotars, footballs and jerseys along with the latest Baby Born, Barbie, gadgets and tech. At home, my own laundry basket always seemed to contain a collection of jerseys, shorts and socks, no matter how often I hung them on the line. GAA was in the very air we breathed and it was impossible to ignore it.

I first met James shortly after coming to Killenaule, when he was a precocious two-year-old. Eight years later, he was a happy, chatty, open and trusting young boy, completely at ease in the familiar consulting room, accompanied by his mother, who sat, redundant, in the background. When I called him from the waiting room he responded immediately and slipped his mobile phone into his pocket, before offering me a cheery 'hello'. I thought him a bit young for a mobile phone, but reminded myself that he was not likely to be coming to me for advice on his use of technology. Before I had a chance to ask him what I could do for him, he addressed me again. 'A great game on Monday night,' he said. 'I bet Joseph was delighted.'

'Did you think so, James?' I asked. For once, I knew what he was talking about and I had to agree; it had been a very exciting game, probably the most exciting I had ever been at. The Killenaule under-12 hurling team had gained a victory over Silvermines to win the county final in Semple Stadium. All of Killenaule were talking about it and all were proud of these young hurlers. All week the stream of people coming in and out of the surgery had been commenting on the match. Winning a county final was a big deal for a club like Killenaule. These young players were a signal of hope. Killenaule was a small pond relative to the towns of Clonmel, Carrick-on-Suir, Thurles or Cahir, with a much smaller shoal of fish to choose from, but that had not deterred them. Winning in Semple Stadium had made it all the sweeter.

On the evening of their victory, a noisy cavalcade of cars drove through the village, in and out of housing estates, hooting and beeping, waving flags jubilantly out of windows and sunroofs, waking sleeping babies, disturbing those who had planned a quiet night in, drawing them to their front doors to offer congratulations to the victors. By the time the tour was completed, a New Holland tractor had been procured and was parked, with trailer attached, outside the Slieveardagh Hotel in the middle of the village. Joe O'Dwyer, an ex-county hurler, was already in position on the trailer as master of ceremonies, a role ideally suited to his gregarious personality, edgy sense of humour and in-depth knowledge of Killenaule hurling. He called each boy in turn and with the adroitness of a professional comedian listed the boy's attributes and contribution to the team. Parents, siblings, aunts, uncles, grannies and grandads looked on proudly from the street.

At one point, I heard Joseph's name being called. 'Joseph Meagher. His father's a doctor, his mother's a doctor, but that hasn't stopped him playing hurling. His determination got him a place on this team and we are glad it did.' Joseph was on the trailer, his face beaming, standing in an excited huddle with his teammates. It was an experience he would never forget. A peak sporting moment.

I turned to James and asked him what I could do for him. He had a sore ear and throat and had not been to school that day. I tried to engage him in chat about himself and his school, while waiting for his prescription to print, but James had no interest in talking about himself. 'How is Joseph getting on in Scoil Ruain?' he asked me, taking control of the conversation, as if he was the adult and I was the child. Scoil Ruain was the secondary school in Killenaule that most of the local children attended.

James's mother interrupted the conversation, telling him not to be delaying the doctor, that I had a lot of people to see and couldn't spend all day talking. I would gladly have spent a while talking to James, but just not about Joseph. At the mention of his name, I experienced an anxious feeling in my chest again, the same feeling that I had been trying to banish all week. 'He is not in Scoil Ruain, James,' I said. 'He has gone to a boarding school in Waterford.'

James looked at me in surprise. 'Waterford!' he exclaimed. 'He's gone all the way to Waterford to school?' He paused for a minute and I remained silent, waiting for him to let it sink in. 'Does he go every day?' he asked.

'Yes,' I replied. 'Every day, James, and he stays there at night as well. It's a boarding school.'

'He's gone to a boarding school. In Waterford. Away from his family,' James exclaimed, his young face darkening with concern and disbelief.

'Yes, James,' I said, fearing I might cry if he kept this up, 'Away from his family.'

'But what did he do?' James asked, emphasising the 'do'.

I laughed when I realised what he was thinking. 'It's not that sort of school. He didn't do anything wrong. It's a nice school, where he will learn lots of new things and make lots of new friends,' I said, feeling glad of the opportunity to think and speak positively about the place. I needed to convince myself more than anyone else that Joseph would be OK.

The day after the county final, I had driven Joseph to Coláiste Na Rinne, or Ring, as it is commonly known, a boarding school in West Waterford, and had left him there to begin a new school year. Because he could not miss the match, he was two days late for the start of school and missed the introductions to the other children and the teachers. As I was leaving the school, feeling extra-guilty that he had missed the first few days and would be immediately at a disadvantage, I was instructed that it was best not to visit him for the first month. I could contact him by phone at a designated time, once a week, but otherwise, I was to stay away and allow him to settle in.

Sending Joseph to Ring had seemed like a good idea when I'd first suggested it to Liam over a year earlier. I had attended an all-Irish boarding school and wanted my children to gain some mastery of the language. I wanted them to be able to listen to Raidió na Gaeltachta and have an idea of what was going on, to hear a poem by Máirtín Ó Díreáin or Máire Mhac an tSaoi and know something of its meaning and appreciate its beauty. Ring offered one year of schooling for children between sixth class in primary school and first year in secondary. I had done my research and anyone that had been there, or had sent their children there, spoke positively of the place. That was all very well in theory, but as I had driven home after bidding Joseph goodbye the previous Monday evening, my heart had been heavy, my eyes had pricked with tears, and I'd wondered what on earth had possessed me to do such a thing.

Joseph's response had been typical of him, neither too excited nor over-anxious, but he was willing to go along with it. Joseph was twelve at this point. He had never been away from home, apart from occasional sleepovers. I had never been separated from him for more than a few days. Living, as we did, without family close by, we operated as a unit. There was, for the most part, just us five. Ours was not a house where kids stayed away from home for days on end with their aunts or uncles. We met every day, all five of us, for breakfast and dinner and slept under the same roof practically every night. At times, all three children and I would be found asleep in the oversized family bed, a leftover habit from the baby years, when I would go to read to them in the late evening. I would start out with Ailshe on one side and Liam Jnr on the other, their homework finished, dinner over, nothing left to do in the busy day but settle down and listen to their own personal audio version of the latest Harry Potter book or *The Chronicles of Narnia*. Later, Joseph would join us, slipping silently under the duvet, keen not to interrupt the story that he himself had already read years before. He would throw his arm casually across his six-year-old brother and eventually nod off with the rest of us. From downstairs I would hear the familiar sounds of Liam moving around the kitchen or turning on the television and feel a sense of complete security. I knew, even as my eyes grew heavy and my words slurred with sleepiness, that these would be among my most treasured memories. All of us well, happy and together.

But I had changed everything. I had sent Joseph away. And it wasn't just me who would miss him. His brother, his sister, his dad, his friends and his teammates – how was he supposed to get along without all of us? I knew how important sport was for Joseph. I knew how much enjoyment he got from playing. Had I ruined his chances of getting back on the hurling team for ever? Uprooted him not only from his family but from a community where he was just beginning to find his feet, just beginning to belong?

I said goodbye to James, still smiling at the thought that he would think Joseph had been sent away for committing some offence, but still bothered by the fact that he had been sent away. Later that evening, I sat in Joseph's vacated room. There were still clothes and books, hurleys and sliotars scattered on every surface. In the corner, amidst the chaos, I saw the bright red of his new football boots, as yet unworn, bought especially for Ring. I pounced on them. 'He's forgotten his boots,' I said to Liam, brandishing them triumphantly in the kitchen. 'He can't manage without his boots.' I had my excuse.

The following Saturday, I was in the car bright and early, merrily making my way to Ring, boots beside me on the passenger seat. I called to reception and, in my best Irish, asked if I could please see Seosamh Ó Meachair. The girl eyed me cautiously. I went on to explain that I was his mother and that I only wanted him for a few minutes because he had forgotten something important. She told me to wait outside. Before long, Joseph appeared, looking happy and healthy and not at all like the homesick waif I had imagined he would have become in the space of a week. He hopped into the passenger seat and reminded me, as if I had forgotten, that I should not be there, before going on to explain that he only had a minute, as they were all going on a tour and he had to get ready. He reminded me he would have to be collected in a couple of weeks, on Saturday at twelve o'clock, and asked if he could get some new clothes in Clonmel on the way home.

I wasn't sure if I was happy or sad, so decided to be happy. The request for new clothes from someone who, until then, would have to be dragged to the shops to replace a tattered tracksuit, made me think that there might be some other females on his radar. Fortunately for both of us, I wasn't quite as important as I'd thought.

Six years later, in 2010, Killenaule won an under-12 county football final. This time, Liam Jnr was on the same trailer, beaming with delight as his brother had before him. The same Joe O'Dwyer introduced the team, but this time there was no reference to being a double doctors' son. Liam had an older brother who had paved the way, flattened a path for him, so that instead of being the doctor's son, he was Joseph Meagher's brother and it was expected that he would be a player.

Later that winter, the team were presented with their medals by their neighbour, role model and future mentor, Declan Fanning, who had just won an All-Ireland medal with Tipperary that year and had been awarded an All-Star hurling medal in 2007. Knowing that Declan, who was born and bred in Killenaule, had gone on to achieve such sporting success made the possibility of playing in Croke Park someday a reality for these young boys. Declan advised the boys that despite his sporting achievements, some of his most treasured and valued memories were of playing for his club alongside his friends and classmates and that they should continue to do this for as long as possible, regardless of winning or losing. 'Keep turning up for training and matches and some of you will, no doubt, play for your county in Croke Park,' he told them. 'But that is not why you should do it. You should do it for the sheer enjoyment of the game, enjoyment that increases the more you play.'

He wasn't wrong about Croke Park. Some of the Killenaule hurlers and footballers who were lucky enough to have Declan's guidance in their formative years were John 'Bubbles' O'Dwyer, Killian O'Dwyer, Joe 'Mouse' O'Dwyer, Jimmy and Paudie Feehan, and they have all gone on to play in Croke Park for their county.

CHAPTER EIGHT

DIVIDED LOYALTIES

I now think that the reason I was not an ardent GAA follower had a lot to do with my experience, or rather lack of experience of GAA as a child. I grew up in Connemara at a time when GAA was a man's sport. On Sundays, when my father and brothers would go to matches, my mother, my sisters and I would remain at home, often peeling apples or chopping rhubarb for the tarts my mother made, which would be devoured by the returning supporters. In my world, it was somehow unseemly for girls to be parading themselves around football pitches. Those who did go were considered notice-boxes who would have been better off at home. I carried this unconscious bias with me into adulthood and despite many attempts by Liam to get me interested in listening to, watching, or going to matches, I only really experienced the highs and lows of hurling and football when my children started to play. I attended their matches with the other mothers and fathers. I shouted from the sidelines, although not as fervently as some of the other mothers, and gradually learned the rules, but I was always in awe of those who could identify their own and everybody else's offspring on the pitch, despite the helmets they wore, and those who knew instinctively when a free was warranted and when it was not. I knew better than to ask any of the other mothers on the sidelines. They were always far too engrossed in the match and would not appreciate my interruptions. Nevertheless, I took my place among the spectators and enjoyed this type of low-key social interaction, where no one expected anything of me. Now that all my children are in their twenties and have left home, I miss these informal opportunities to connect with other mothers and fathers, to discuss the banalities of the weather, the too-long summer holidays, the fact of not being able to go anywhere because there was sure to be a match. But behind the mock complaining was gratitude for the opportunity our children had to play team sports and an appreciation for the people who gave voluntarily of their time to make this happen.

My children liked me to see them play, but they had one rule that I was not to breach. NEVER, EVER set foot on the pitch when they were playing a match. 'But what if you get injured and fall down and don't get up?' I asked one day. 'I can hardly just sit on the sideline and do nothing.' But they were adamant. If a doctor was needed, then I should wait to be called by one of the officials. There were mammies who occasionally went on to the pitch when their offspring took a slap or fell down inexplicably. If I ever did this, I would be banned from matches indefinitely. I didn't protest, but thought silently that I would decide my own level of restraint on that one.

A few years earlier, in 2001, Tipperary and Galway had been due to play in the All-Ireland hurling final. A parcel arrived addressed to me, from my brother, Gerry. In it was a very large Galway flag, with a note pinned to it, 'Up Galway'. I had a dilemma. I knew my children, then aged nine, seven and three, all staunch Tipperary supporters, would never let me get away with raising that flag anywhere near our house – but I couldn't not support Galway. I hid it away for a couple of days, while figuring out what to do.

Eventually, I decided to raise the flag. I didn't tell anyone, just got up early on the Saturday morning before the match, appropriated a pole from an old Mayo flag that had belonged to Liam and that had been abandoned in the shed, attached the Galway flag and stuck it in the wire of the fence right outside the kitchen window. I figured this was a compromise of sorts. The flag could not be seen by passers-by on the road. It would only be evident to visitors to the house. I thought I might get away with that.

A little while later, the three sleepy heads arose and, as was their habit, settled themselves in the sitting room to watch Saturday morning television. Eventually, they emerged into the kitchen, where I was sitting at the table reading a magazine. For the next few minutes, the only sounds were those of spoons on bowls and the crunching of cereal until all of a sudden, Joseph dropped his spoon, sending milk spattering all over the table, pushed his chair back and dashed to the window. He stared, speechless, at the flag flapping gently in the breeze, before turning to me with an accusatory look and I knew I had done a terrible thing. 'Mum, did you do that?' he asked, once he'd recovered his speech, his childish face a mixture of disbelief and betrayal.

I went on the offensive. 'I might have,' I replied. 'What if I did?'

He managed to compose himself enough to say that the flying of a Galway flag anywhere near our house was totally unacceptable. How could I not know that? He called on his siblings to support him. His father had mysteriously disappeared, although I could have sworn that he was in the kitchen earlier and was definitely somewhere within earshot. By then, Ailshe and Liam Jnr were also indignant and agreed with their brother that I should take the flag down at once.

'I can hang a flag outside my house if I want,' I asserted.

'Take it down, Mum,' Joseph pleaded. 'You probably won't even watch the match. We can't have a Galway flag outside our house. You don't even follow GAA. I bet you can't even name one Galway hurler.'

'I can so,' I said, naming Joe Rabbitte, the 'Fox-chaser,' the only one I knew. I gave Joseph a smug smile, feeling quite pleased with myself. I didn't add that everybody knew Joe Rabbitte, who had earned his nickname after Mícheál Ó Muircheartaigh's famous commentary on a match where Joe had chased the Tipperary player Pat Fox down the pitch. 'I've seen it all now. A Rabitte chasing a Fox around Croke Park.'

'But I've seen you read a book in Croke Park, the last time Dad brought you with us,' Joseph retorted. 'That's how much interest you had in the match.'

'That's not true,' I replied. I explained to him that I had never read a book during a match. Maybe while waiting for it to start, or at half-time, but never during. 'Fair's fair,' I said. 'I support Tipperary against every other team except Galway and if I want to put up a flag outside my own house, I should be able to do so.'

I was beginning to convince myself that I really did want the flag flying. I decided that that was a good time to exit and escaped to do the weekly shopping, leaving three cross faces behind, pleading with their dad, who had reappeared and who could honestly say he had no knowledge of the offending flag, to 'do something'.

'And don't anyone touch that flag while I'm gone,' I called from the hall door, before pulling it closed behind me. When I returned a few hours later, it was to a very different atmosphere. Liam Jnr ran out to me, his face beaming. 'Well, what are you so happy about?' I asked.

'Nothing,' he replied, but couldn't stop grinning.

'Have ye taken down my flag?' I asked, wondering if he had been sent to break the news to me, as he was the one I was least likely to get cross with.

'No,' he said, barely able to contain himself, as he took my hand and led me towards the fence. Eventually, I spotted the source of his glee. I could no longer see the Galway flag, but not because it had been taken down, simply because it was now surrounded by four even bigger Tipperary flags. I had to admit defeat. I never found out whose idea it was or where they got the flags in the short time that I was away and to this day nobody will tell me. The following day, Tipperary had another victory when they beat Galway in the All-Ireland hurling final.

It seemed that no matter how hard I tried and no matter how much exposure to the GAA I got, I was destined never to become an expert in that particular field. Not so many years ago, while heading to the kitchen for a hard-earned cup of tea after morning surgery, I noticed Angela, the secretary at the time, talking to a tall, handsome young man at the reception desk. He was dressed in a suit and was leaning on the counter in a relaxed but engaging manner. As I passed by, I heard her say, 'The doctors here do not see reps. They haven't done so for years.'

It was true that Liam and I had decided not to see representatives from drug companies in our surgery. This was due to a combination of there being too many reps on the road and some reps forgetting to turn up for appointments. It was not an easy decision to make and we deliberated over it for some time, before concluding that it was probably best to say no to all new reps. Those who had been coming regularly would go on a 'whitelist' and we would continue to see them. So it was unusual for a rep to cold-call to the surgery and hearing Angela explain the situation made me feel a little guilty. I still had trouble saying 'no' to lots of requests.

The man told Angela his name, which didn't sound familiar, and asked if he could leave his card. To assuage my guilt and because

I felt it would be rude not to go and explain myself, seeing as he knew I was lurking in the kitchen, I stepped into the reception area and introduced myself. I explained our policy regarding reps and briefly outlined why we had come to this decision. He said he understood and apologised if anyone from his company had ever missed a pre-booked appointment. He said he would leave his card anyway and asked if we would mind contacting him if we decided at any date in the future to change our policy. I said I would. We shook hands and he went reluctantly towards the door.

He had only just left when, Bernie, our nurse, who had been in her own room with the door open, rushed into the waiting room and peered out the door after him. 'Girls,' she said, craning her neck to get a look into the car park. 'Did that man say his name was Henry Shefflin?'

Angela looked down at the card in her hand and read the name. 'Henry Shefflin,' she said. 'Yes, you're right. Do you know him?'

Bernie looked at us both in shocked disbelief. 'Henry Shefflin,' she exclaimed. Don't tell me ye don't know Henry Shefflin? Just about the most famous hurler in the country. How could ye not recognise Henry Shefflin?'

Now that she had repeated it a few times, the name did ring a bell.

Bernie was still standing, looking flabbergasted. 'It's his autograph you should have been getting,' she said to me, 'not sending him away because you don't see reps. Wait until Liam hears that ye turned away Henry Shefflin.'

'Well, I was only doing my job,' Angela replied. 'We do have a policy and I was only following it.'

'I was being just and fair and treating everybody the same,' I attempted in my defence.

'Henry Shefflin is not everybody,' Bernie replied, exasperated. 'He is not the same as anyone else. He is a legend. I've lost count of how many All-Ireland titles he has and he's been hurler of the year at least twice, if not three times. Have you any idea how excited people would be to see Henry Shefflin in the waiting room? There would be a queue up to the shop for photographs.' She retired to her room, shaking her head in disgust and disbelief.

I looked at Angela. 'I suppose we should really have recognised him,' I said, 'but I don't watch that much GAA and even when I do, they are wearing helmets. I don't even recognise my own children when they are wearing them.' I retreated to my consulting room feeling a bit deflated. My kids would never forgive me if they ever heard that I had turned away the most famous hurler in the country. I would certainly never be allowed to fly another Galway flag. I decided that that was one story I would not be sharing around the dinner table.

CHAPTER NINE

'DOING A LOCUM'

Holidays are a frequent topic of conversation at any gathering of country GPs, but there are no questions like, 'Where did you go?' and 'What was it like?' or long descriptions of far-flung exotic places, followed by shared holiday photographs. No tips on family resorts, romantic hideaways or the most interesting European city break. No, these conversations will be all about locums. 'Did you find one?' 'Where did you find one?' 'What were they like and are they still available?' The holiday destinations are secondary: the most challenging part of arranging holidays is finding someone to look after the practice when you go. Those who can manage to do that with relative ease are held in awe by those of us who frequently cannot.

Every GP has what I call the 'locum disaster stories', where the doctor failed to appear, arrived late, fought with everyone once they were there and had to leave early because of a family crisis. Alongside this are tales of excellent doctors who looked after not only the surgery and the house, but the dog, cat and, in extreme circumstances, the children as well. We had experiences of both kinds, but every year was the same, with us not knowing if we would get a locum or not, because all types of locum were in short supply. This situation still exists today, especially for rural practices like ours. We still deal with it in the same way: optimistically blocking off the desired weeks' leave, asking around, checking the locum agencies and hoping for the best.

When the children were young, every summer we would return to my native Renvyle, where my parents, aunts, uncles and some of my siblings still lived. As well as reconnecting with family, it felt good to spend time among the Twelve Bens and the bog and grasslands of Connemara. I wanted my children to know that they had a special link with this magical place, even if I had chosen not to live there. I wanted them to know it as another home, where people knew their names and their ancestry. In the Connemara Caravan and Camping Park on Lettergesh beach we had our very own mobile home that we could return to at will and it was there we were heading on a sunny Saturday in July 1999, having loaded the car, closed up the house and, miraculously, secured a locum.

In the car, I went through a mental checklist of all the tasks that had absolutely needed to be completed before we left and found that, for once, they had all been done. As is my habit, not being satisfied with having completed the absolutely necessary tasks, I went through another checklist of tasks that ideally should have been done and, of course, I wasn't long finding one. 'We probably should have fixed that door handle before we left,' I said, more to myself than to Liam, who was happily driving west, already completely switched off from work and Killenaule.

'Forget about it,' he said. The fact that the handle on the door of his consulting room was faulty was a detail he did not need to be reminded of as he set off on his holidays. He added that I should stop worrying about the surgery: we would be back there soon enough and would have plenty of opportunity to sort out anything that needed sorting.

Of course, the best way to keep thinking about something is to try not to think about it, so I returned to my ruminations.

Sometimes, when the door was closed from the inside, the door handle would detach, meaning that the door could not be opened from either the inside or the outside, until the handle was manoeuvred back on again. Liam, Bridget and I had become experts at working around this problem, but this was not an ideal situation for a locum, especially not Dr Mick Murphy, the doctor we had left in charge, who had vast experience of dealing with patients, but was not in any way mechanically minded.

But we were going on holidays and Liam was right: I needed to stop thinking about the surgery. So, I turned my thoughts to our holiday and to what we would do when we got there. One of my favourite things to do as a teenager would be to take my bicycle the three miles from our house in Derryherbert, through Tullycross, down the Gurteen Road, past the pink cottage on the right, then left at the T-junction and on to the shoreline. There, I would abandon the bicycle on the smooth grey stones and pick my way over the rocks to the pier, where I would sit for a while and savour the sights and sounds of the sea: white caps or a calm swell, the tideline littered with spume and the waves lapping against the dark grey of the pier wall. From there, I would cross the little river to the beach, Trá Na mBan, before continuing up and over the headland, where I would get my first view of Renvyle Beach Caravan and Camping Park, with its collection of coloured caravans, tents and outdoor furniture. I would not venture near the caravan park; instead, I would climb the fence and make my way down onto White Strand, as we always called Renvyle beach, where the pristine sand lay undisturbed by footprints, making me loath to sully it with my own. If it was summer, I would take off my shoes and walk along the water's edge, leaving my footprints to disappear behind me as I went. My destination was Renvyle House Hotel, but only because that was as far as I could walk on the peninsula. Once I got there, I would simply turn around and do the whole journey back again, retrieving my bicycle and setting off for home. Thinking about how I would soon be able to do this again wiped all thoughts of faulty door handles, locums and patients from my mind.

My thoughts were disturbed by Joseph, looking up from the latest Harry Potter book in the back of the car, asking if we would be in Renvyle in time to go jumping off the pier that evening.

'It depends on the tides,' I said. 'If the tide is right, then we will go.'

Nowadays, Ailshe or Liam would check the tides on their phone, but in those pre-internet and smartphone days, we just had to wait until we got to the sea. Each day of the holidays, in sunshine or rain, we would check the tides and congregate at Tully pier with other like-minded families, to jump off the high wall. I was a reluctant swimmer. I loved being in the water and loved getting out, but I hated getting in, so I never jumped off the pier. I usually watched with a mixture of nervousness, admiration and envy as Liam and the kids climbed up onto the high wall and balanced themselves on the top before leaping into the deep, dark water. They would shriek with delight as they jumped, anticipating the splash as they landed. I would watch the swirling water with anticipation until they reappeared, eyes tightly closed, pushing the hair off their faces, swimming to the rope that someone had tied to the stone pillar, before pulling themselves up to do it all over again. We had a rule, though. They could only jump off the pier if Liam was with them. There was only so much excitement a mother could witness.

My thoughts returned to the surgery and to the doctor we had asked to be our locum. Dr Michael Murphy had worked as a GP for over forty years and was semi-retired from his own practice, which was also in Killenaule. He was a tidy figure of a man of medium height, with a full head of grey hair, who always dressed in a suit, shirt and tie. He lived with Ena, his wife and right-hand woman. They were always together, both inside and outside the surgery. By the time we got to know them, their children were long since grown and had left home. For most of his forty years in Killenaule, Dr Murphy would be in his surgery every day except Wednesday, and available to his patients every night at his home. On Wednesdays, he and Ena went to Dublin, where they would visit their grown-up children. On arriving back home at nine o'clock at night there would frequently be a queue of patients outside their door. 'We knew you would be back, Doctor. So we thought we would hang on, rather than go to Doctor Stokes in Fethard,' one of them would say.

He would tend to them without a murmur of complaint.

When Liam explained to him that we were working a one-weekend-in-four, out-of-hours rota with the GPs in Ballingarry and Fethard, and that all of us were willing to include his patients in that out-of-hours cover, he was overcome. He found it difficult to comprehend that he could simply put on his answering machine in the evening, or indeed any time that he did not want to be disturbed, and come and go as he pleased. 'You mean, I can just switch the phone to you and you will all cover my patients in the evenings and at weekends?'

'Yes,' Liam said, explaining that we were on call anyway and a few more patients would not make any difference. Every Sunday evening Liam was on call, Dr Murphy would ring to check if any of his patients had needed attention. These Sunday evening telephone conversations usually extended to much more than queries about patients.

'Do you know?' he said once to Liam. 'I haven't been inside a bank since I came back to Ireland from the Channel Islands and that's over thirty years ago.' This was undoubtedly true, as Ena did all the banking and shopping. It was Ena who arranged meetings with the accountant, solicitor, or home maintenance people and

Ena who organised their social calendar, such as it was. Dr Murphy attended to his patients, studied medical books and journals and maintained a keen interest in all things related to medicine. His experience of country practice showed how much things had changed over the years. He recounted tales of delivering babies on his examination couch, identifying the body of a young man who had lost his life in the Ballingarry coal mines and doing endless house calls during the flu pandemic of 1968, sometimes getting there only to pronounce yet another person dead. He never lost his interest in people and the illnesses they develop.

'Would you mind seeing me today, Doctor?' a patient of his asked me one day. 'I just don't have time to see Doctor Murphy.'

'What do you mean?' I asked, 'Is he very busy?'

'Oh, no, he's not, but that's the problem. He is not busy at all, so he will keep me all day chatting.'

This was not a common complaint about doctors, but it demonstrated how much Dr Murphy enjoyed his work, that in his last years of practice he could make two or three patients last a whole morning.

Bridget had offered Dr Murphy a choice of consulting rooms to work in while he was covering our holidays and he had chosen Liam's. Locums seemed to prefer Liam's room to mine: I thought this might be because most of the replacement doctors were male and my room was more of a lady doctor's room, with children's paintings on the walls and all sorts of suspicious-looking 'women's things' on the trolley at the end of the couch. It might have been that my room was just too tidy. They might have been afraid of disturbing the order, of not putting things back in their rightful place. Liam's room did not have rightful places for things, despite the fact that I sometimes went in there and reordered all his shelves and drawers, even sticking labels on containers in the hope that, eventually, the order would be maintained. Liam only noticed that I had been in when he couldn't find something and had to ask me, with a mixture of irritation and resignation, if I had been tidying again. He claimed he had a perfectly adequate sorting and filing system, but that is one thing we have never agreed on. I would frequently agree not to interfere with his room and he would agree to maintain some sort of order and this truce would last another three months or so, until I could not resist imposing my order once again.

Liam had tidied his room before leaving, but I would have preferred Dr Murphy to work from my room, as I was fearful that he would have trouble with the faulty door handle. As it turned out I was right.

As Bridget recounted the story on our return, it was about mid-way through his first morning as locum and Dr Murphy decided to have a cigarette break. He told the patients in the waiting room that he would be with them shortly, went back into the consulting room and closed the door. As expected, the handle came off in his hand. He left it aside and had his cigarette, but when he tried to put it back on again, he could not manage it. Bridget heard banging and shouting from inside the room, but when she tried to get in, she found that as the central spindle of the handle had come out, turning the handle on the outside of the door had no effect.

Bridget was naturally reserved and efficient and would not voluntarily draw attention to herself. She was happiest behind the counter in reception, where people could not invade her personal space, but that morning, she found herself shouting through the door, guiding Dr Murphy through the process of reattaching the handle, in full view and well within earshot of all the people in the waiting room. There was no way Dr Murphy could get the handle back on the door. He was stuck inside the room and it was only day one of his two-week locum.

Bridget gave up on the instructions and went outside, to see if there was any way of getting in through a window. She knew that if she got into the room, she would manage to open the door. The surgery windows were big, but only the top third could actually be opened, allowing just about enough space for a small child to fit through. Nonetheless, Bridget estimated that she was probably slim enough to negotiate it. She went back to the waiting room to get a chair to climb on to. A middle-aged man sprang up help her and she felt she could not spurn his chivalry.

The particular window that had the easiest access to Dr Murphy's room was in full view of the car park and many of the cars were occupied with relatives waiting to take people home after their consultation. By then, all of the waiting room patients had followed Bridget and her helper outside. The audience grew. The relatives got out of their cars and wanted to know what the trouble was. Between fifteen and twenty people crowded around Bridget, looking at her, looking at the window, nodding or shaking their heads, depending on whether they thought she would, or would not, fit through the window. She eventually got in, opened the door and she and Dr Murphy emerged, to a round of applause from the crowd.

'You must have been cursing us for not getting the handle fixed,' I said, when she had finished her story on our first day back after our holidays. I could not resist throwing Liam an 'I told you so' look, while feeling guilty that I had not insisted that the door be fixed before we left.

'So, who was the lucky guy who got to give you a leg-up?' Liam asked. 'I'm sure there were a lot of volunteers.'

Bridget shot him a look that said there was no one putting a hand anywhere near her. Either she got in there by herself, or she was not going in at all.

'And how did Doctor Murphy cope with all this stress?' I asked.

'He wasn't a bit bothered,' Bridget replied. 'He was sitting back in the chair, reading one of Liam's medical journals, smoking away, not a care in the world.'

Bridget lost no time moving Dr Murphy into my consulting room and by the time we returned, the door had been fixed. One of the patients who had been in the waiting room that day knew a man, who had the job done in minutes.

Dr Murphy has since passed away. As is the case with a lot of medical professionals, when he was told he had terminal cancer, he chose not to go to hospital and declined the invasive tests and aggressive treatments that might have prolonged his life, but that would certainly have decreased the quality of the time he had left. Liam managed his care and he remained well and in good form until a couple of days before he died. Ena is still a frequent visitor to our house. From her usual place at the kitchen table, she often admonishes me for working too hard, reminds me that my husband is 'a gift from God' and bestows heaps of praise on my children, who can do no wrong in her eyes.

One day recently, I reminded her of the time that Mick had done our locum and got locked in the consulting room. She had no memory of it, but laughed as she agreed that that would be typical of Mick. 'We were so foolish, weren't we?' she said. 'Working all those hours. We'd be like children getting out of school if we got a couple of hours off to go out to dinner in Cashel or Fethard. It was crazy, but Mick never complained. He was such a patient man.'

'He must have been,' I replied, 'but sure, he had you, Ena. It was easy for him to be patient. Just like Liam, there,' I joked. I had just joined her at the kitchen table, where she was sitting watching Liam, who had taken a roast out of the oven and was checking the potatoes on the hob. He was wearing a blue butcher's-style apron that Ailshe had bought him a few months earlier. 'A good wife makes anything bearable,' I said.

Ena looked at me with raised eyebrows. 'A good husband is what you got,' she said. 'There is no chance that you would ever have found Mick Murphy in the kitchen checking potatoes, or even making a cup of tea. I honestly believe he did not even know how to turn on the cooker.'

'The poor man,' Liam said. 'You mean you never showed him how?'

Ena laughed and I thought how much our lives, so similar in many ways, were also very different. Middle-of-the-night call-outs, late-evening surgeries and forty-eight-hour weekend shifts are thankfully a thing of the past for most GPs; GP's wives or husbands do not have to stay home all the time to answer the phone, or give up a potential career, as Ena, a qualified radiographer, had done, in order to facilitate a partner's practice. And most husbands nowadays know their way around the kitchen – but finding a locum for holiday or sick leave is still a source of stress for many.

CHAPTER TEN

THE ART OF SAYING NO

Nora was a tall, thin woman, slightly bent at the waist, with a head of wiry grey hair, supported on a thin neck that jutted out in front of her when she walked. As a medical student, I had heard this described as 'bird-like posture' by a rheumatologist in Galway. It was not a universally recognised medical term, but it described Nora perfectly. As she walked, she leaned heavily on her stick and with each step her body moved from side to side, as well as forward. As a result, she made slow progress. Before ever she had an X-ray, it was obvious that she had osteoarthritis of her hips.

Once she was sitting comfortably in my consultation room, she asked me again, as she had many times previously, for 'something for the pains'.

'Nora,' I replied, my voice inclined to match the unvaried monotony of her tone, my body language automatically mirroring hers, 'the only way to get rid of those pains is to have a hip operation. Otherwise, paracetamol is the safest treatment for you, but that doesn't seem to work.'

'At my age, Doctor, I'm not going to have an operation,' she said with a mixture of stoicism and stubbornness. 'I suppose I will just have to put up with it, so.'

I felt sorry for Nora. Sorry that I could not offer anything more for her pain. Sorry that she would not have an operation. I wondered, if she were my grandmother, what I would have wanted her to do. I would probably still have urged her towards an operation. Hip operations usually have a good outcome, even in someone like Nora, who, despite being in her mid-eighties, was otherwise healthy.

'Well, you are on the waiting list, Nora,' I said. 'So, if you get called, I think you should at least go and talk to the specialist. They won't do an operation if they think you are not fit, but it is not good for you to be in pain all the time.' I stopped talking then, aware that we had already had this conversation more than once and that Nora was no longer listening. She was rummaging in the big shopping bag that she always carried with her. I sat back and waited. I figured I had been caught again. Whatever she produced from the bag was going to be the real reason she came in: a form for the council applying for new windows, a medical certificate to say she was fit to go to Lourdes, a letter to say she was still alive, so that she could continue to receive her UK pension.

I noticed that whenever a patient wanted me to do something that was not strictly what a doctor should be doing, they usually tested me first by presenting a clinical problem – a pain, an ache or a cough. Once on familiar territory, they would gauge my mood, gently leading me to the point where they would produce the offending document with an air of shared frustration at the bureaucrats who deemed this necessary.

On this occasion, I was wrong. Nora handed me a package, a brown Dunnes Stores paper bag, rolled over at the top so that I could not see what was in it. She passed it to me with the same doleful expression she always wore. 'I thought your daughter would like this,' she said. 'I saw it in the little charity shop in Killenaule and I thought of her.'

I straightened up and took the package, caught completely off guard, ashamed of my earlier cynicism. It wasn't unusual for people to give gifts at Christmas, even though I did not encourage or expect it, but it was only the middle of summer. 'Thank you, Nora,' I said. 'That's very kind of you, but you shouldn't have.'

'It's only a little something,' she said. 'You can look, if you like. She might like to take it on her holidays.'

I opened the bag and withdrew a small, brown leopard-print messenger bag, with splashes of fuchsia pink on the outside and sparkles on the handle. It could have been for a child or adult, it was hard to tell. It had a charity shop smell, musty with a hint of mothballs. 'Thank you, Nora,' I said again. 'It's lovely. She will be chuffed. It's definitely the sort of thing she likes.'

I was baffled. Why Nora would have been reminded of Ailshe when she'd seen the bag, I wondered. I didn't even know that she knew her. At ten, Ailshe was a conspicuous-looking child, with white-blonde hair, blue eyes and a pretty, endearing face. It was difficult not to notice her, even in a crowd in the church or at school events. But compared to her friend Gráinne, an outgoing bubbly extrovert, Ailshe was quiet and circumspect, kept herself to herself and listened more than she spoke. I had no idea why Nora would have singled her out for a gift, but my mood lifted, my earlier cynicism vanished and I felt happy that this lady, living alone, her own grandchildren long since grown and living abroad, would get joy from giving to my child.

Ailshe knew exactly who I was talking about when I gave her the bag later that evening. 'I often meet her at the surgery,' she said, 'and she always says hello.' Nora had a habit of calling to the surgery without an appointment, at around midday, when she expected I had finished all my morning appointments and that she could be seen straight away. I had tried to discourage this, but Nora was beyond training and so I usually just saw her and warned her not to tell anyone else. Ailshe, when she was on holiday from school, also had a habit of popping in to see me at around this time, just to see that I was where I was supposed to be and that I would be home for lunch, as well as to bring me up to speed with the agenda that she had planned for us for the afternoon. The two regularly bumped into each other in this manner. 'Birds of a feather,' I thought. They both know how to make sure they get what they want.

Nora did not get a call to the orthopaedic clinic to have her hip assessed, so she continued to consult me, in the hope that there was something new on the market that would alleviate her pains. My response was always the same: what she really needed was a new hip. Her mobility was decreasing, her sleep was disturbed and she was losing weight, but her enthusiasm for human connection and for life in general did not show any signs of waning.

A couple of months after Nora had given me the gift, at the end of a consultation, as I held the door open for her to leave, she produced a document from her ever-present shopping bag. 'I'll leave this with you,' she said. 'You might put a signature on it, in your own time.'

I automatically took a step back, in order to put some distance between me and the offending document. I had no idea what it was, but anything anyone wanted me to do 'in my own time' was usually not good. I often wondered what people meant exactly when they said this. Did they think that that the time they were with me was their time? That the time they were not with me was my time and I should use it for these menial tasks, rather than waste their time?

I was in a bit of a mood. It was the end of a busy morning and I was in need of my lunch. 'What is it, Nora?' I asked, still not taking it from her. I was well aware of the game we were playing. Once this form was in my possession, it was my responsibility to complete it satisfactorily. I had already warned Bridget never to take a form from anyone and let them walk away. If I was going to have to spend time filling something out, then the least the patient could do was be there to witness me doing it. At least that way, no one could later quibble with what I had written on it.

'It's my driver's licence,' she said. 'Can you believe, I have to have it signed every year now? Sure, it's no length since I did it before. I'll pick it up next week, Doctor. I don't want to rush you now.'

'You know I can't just put a signature on it, Nora. I have to check your eyesight and do a medical check to make sure that you are safe to drive. That's what my signature means. I'm sorry, but you will have to book another appointment.'

'Oh, alright,' she said in her low, monotonous tone. 'But there's nothing wrong with my eyes. And I only do short journeys in and out of the town and maybe to Fethard on a Friday.'

I was still holding the door open for her and the few patients left in the waiting room were looking in, anxious for her to leave so that they could have their turn. They had been delayed long enough.

'Can you do it now?' she asked, as a last-ditch effort. 'I'm not in any rush today.'

'I'm sorry, Nora,' I said. 'I still have a few people to see and we have already spent a fair bit of time going through your other problems. Another day, if you don't mind.' She left, saying she would see me the following week. I knew that there was a chance that I would not be able to put my signature on that document and that would mean that Nora could no longer drive. It was not a consultation I was looking forward to.

As expected, one week later I was trying to explain to Nora that her eyesight was not good enough for me to sign the form. She would have to stop driving. 'I'm sorry, Nora,' I said. 'I'm afraid I can't sign it this time. Your eyesight is not good enough to keep you, or others, safe if you are driving.'

'But, Doctor, I can see fine. I can see those sheep out there at the far end of the field,' she said, looking over my right shoulder through the window behind me. 'And when I stand at my own kitchen window at home, I can see the cat in the bushes at the far end of the garden. I just can't make out the letters on that chart. I never was one for letters.'

I didn't respond. Her eyesight was not anywhere near the required standard for driving.

'If you give me that chart, I will take it home and practise it,' she went on, as if she had just found the solution. 'I'm sure I will read it fine, if you want to do it again.'

'I can't do that, Nora. This chart is to test your eyesight, not your memory. I'm quite sure there is nothing wrong with your memory. Maybe once you get your cataracts done, I can re-test you. You might be OK then,' I said, to soften the blow. Nora was also on a waiting list for cataract operations, but there was also a long waiting list for this procedure. I knew that if Nora stopped driving even for a short time, she was likely to lose confidence and not drive again. Nevertheless, I was not responsible for the waiting lists and nobody would thank me if Nora injured herself or somebody else on the road while she was waiting.

I expected her to be upset, to protest that she would only do short journeys, but she was grudgingly accepting. We had a long history of mutual respect and I'm sure that helped her to know that I only had her best interests at heart and so she accepted my decision, despite her disappointment.

Nowadays, there are lots of sophisticated specialist tests that can be done, including on- and off-road assessments to test reaction times, motor strength and cognitive function, but in those days the decision to renew the driver's licence was the responsibility of the GP and was always something of a grey area. The topic had come up at a GP educational meeting one evening and an older GP offered his solution. 'What I do is, I take the form and tell them to leave it with me, that I will get back to them in a week or so. I make sure to get out to the local pub at least one night in the week and make discreet enquiries about so-and-so's driving. If the general consensus is that it is OK, then I go ahead and sign. If it causes any raised eyebrows or stories of near-misses, I won't.'

'Sure, you have to ask around,' another experienced GP interjected, surprised that this method of community consensus was news to us young ones. 'You can't be expected to know who is and who isn't safe to be on the road.'

Saying 'no' to people is always difficult, even though it is an almost daily requirement. Some requests are easier to refuse than others, because they involve doing something that does not constitute good medical practice, such as requests for sleeping tablets or sick notes for people who are not actually sick and who would be better off getting back into the workplace. Other requests are more difficult to refuse, because even though I know they are a waste of time, the patient has been sent to me by someone else who has told them that a letter or a phone call from me will get them what they want. These include requests to the county council for home improvements, or letters to consultants to expedite appointments and move them up the waiting list. But in my practice, the most difficult request of all to refuse is a signature on a fitness-to-drive certificate. Not being able to drive in a place like Killenaule can quickly lead to social isolation and loneliness and have a very negative effect on a person's health. Of course, there is Ring-a-Link, the voluntary minibus service, as well as taxis and the daily bus from Thurles to Clonmel and back again, which comes through Killenaule, but there is nothing like being able to drive your own car, going where you want to go, when you decide you want to go there.

Now, at our consultation, Nora was talking again, in the same resigned and unenthusiastic tone. 'I suppose I have been lucky to be driving until now and you have to do your job.'

'But how will you manage to get around?' I asked, feeling guilty, even though it was not my fault.

'Oh, I'll manage,' she said. 'I always do. ' And she shuffled out of the surgery, stick in one hand and handbag in the other, head jutting out in front of her, muttering a sorrowful goodbye to the other patients in the waiting room as she went.

One day, a month or so later, while driving the seven miles from Killenaule to Fethard, past Coolmore Stud, with its manicured roadside lawns, beech hedges and rows of native Irish trees, I spotted a lone figure standing at the roadside, stick in one hand, shopping bag on the road beside her, her left thumb raised in a typical hitchhiker pose. There was no doubting that figure. It was Nora. I pulled over and leaned across the seat, opening the passenger door for her. 'Hello, Nora,' I called.

She shuffled over to the door, eased her way into the car, settled herself in and closed the door. Only then did she look to see who was driving. 'Who have I here?' she asked, leaning over towards me and peering into my face.

'It's me, Nora,' I said. 'Doctor Gannon.'

'Oh, that's great,' she said. 'Are you going to Fethard?'

'I am,' I replied. 'I have to do a quick run into the chemist.'

'Good, good,' she said, more to herself than to me. 'I have to go in to the solicitor. I have a bit of business to do. It's hard to go anywhere now that I am not driving.'

'Well, I can drop you there,' I said, delighted that I could be of some use, guilt resurging once more with the mention of her not driving.

'I have a bit of shopping to do in the supermarket, as well,' she said, without looking at me. 'Would you be able to drop me there afterwards? I only have a few things to get. I won't be long.'

'Well, I just came out between surgeries to pick up a few things from the chemist. I have a surgery starting in half an hour,' I replied.

'Oh, don't worry,' she said, I'll tell the solicitor you are in a hurry. I'll make sure she sees me straight away.'

I was in deeper than I expected. Even out of the surgery, I was no match for Nora. 'Have you an appointment with the solicitor?' I asked, knowing I should not even be entertaining the possibility of waiting for her while she got all her errands done. I knew the pace she moved at and she was no Concorde. Also, I was not lying when I said I had a surgery in half an hour. On the other hand, what could I do? I couldn't just abandon her in Fethard.

'I never make an appointment,' Nora explained. 'It's not the same as the surgery. You just go in and wait, but if I tell her the doctor is waiting for me and you have to get back straight away, I'm sure she will see me fairly quickly.'

I thought to myself that even though she was supposed to make an appointment in the surgery, she never did, but I had advised her not to tell anyone about it, so I suppose I should have been grateful that she at least paid lip-service to the practice. Nevertheless, I wondered if the solicitor really did operate a walk-in service.

Once in Fethard, we pulled up outside the solicitor's office and I hopped out and went around to open the door for Nora. 'I'll be back in a few minutes,' I said, 'and if you are ready, I will pick you up and I might just have time to wait for you while you get a few things in the shop.'

As I closed the car door after her, she straightened herself up and headed towards the door to the solicitor's office. Then she turned to me. 'Oh, Doctor, the door is closed,' she said. 'Her girl will be in there though. If you knock on the window there for me, she will let you in.'

I don't want to go in, I thought. I don't want to knock on the window. If the door is closed, then it's closed for a reason.

Nora was making steady progress towards the door. She noticed my reluctance. 'Just a tap on that window there and she will come out and open the door,' she repeated, as if I had not heard her the first time.

I couldn't just walk away, so I looked in the window and spotted a girl I did not know, because I'd never been to that solicitor's office, sitting inside. I knocked gently and the girl looked up at me quizzically. I pointed towards Nora, who was standing at the door, waiting to be let in, but out of view of the girl. The girl rose and came over to the window, looking sideways, trying to make sense of my gesticulations. Finally, she gave in and opened the door.

'Hello, Nora,' she said, with that same look that I had given Nora so many times, when she had turned up at the surgery without notice. 'Are you looking to make an appointment?'

Nora put on her most sorrowful voice. 'I'm with the doctor,' she said, nodding in my direction. 'And she has to get back to her surgery fairly soon, so I wonder if I could be seen straight away. I won't be long.'

I didn't know whether to go or stay. The girl looked at me for an explanation, but I had none to give. I turned to Nora. 'I'm sorry, Nora,' I said, 'I really can't stay to bring you home if you have to wait for the solicitor and then get your shopping. I will have people waiting for me and I really need to get my things and go back.'

The solicitor's secretary was much better at 'no' than I was. 'I have people waiting already,' she said to both of us. 'I can't ask them to let you in first.'

'Will they be long?' asked Nora.

'I have no idea,' the secretary replied. 'It all depends on what they want.' The secretary was unapologetic. That's just the way it was. I could learn a thing or two from her, I thought.

I have often thought that there is too high a value put on empathy at the expense of assertiveness throughout medical training. Always putting ourselves in other people's shoes can tie us up in knots and leave us powerless in the presence of pros like Nora. Now, I took the secretary's example. 'I'll leave you to it, Nora,' I said. 'I'm sure you will get someone to take you home.'

Completely unabashed, Nora was already making her way into the hallway, pushing open the door to the waiting room. She sat next to a man she seemed to recognise. 'Are you going to Killenaule when you finish here?' she asked him.

'Looks like she has her lift home,' I said to the secretary, with a smile that said, 'I don't think even you will get yourself out of this one.' The secretary did not seem to hear me or to notice that I was leaving. She simply watched as Nora settled herself in the waiting room.

Nora had got her way again. She might be off the road, but she was not off her stride. If anything, she was even more resourceful and determined than ever.

CHAPTER ELEVEN

A DELICATE MATTER

I often wonder what my life would have been like if I had never learned to read, as books have played such a big part in directing the course of my life. I have no doubt that it was the timely reading of *The Politics of Breastfeeding* by Gabrielle Palmer when Joseph was four months old that influenced me to breastfeed my three children for much longer than I otherwise would. The book outlined the harm done to mothers and babies globally for the sake of profit by the formula companies and the methods they use to convince society that formula feeding is necessary and beneficial. Long before I finished it, I vowed never to buy a tin of infant formula milk.

It was the words of a famous physician, Dr William Osler, that influenced me to apply to the University of Limerick Graduate Entry Medical School for a job as a clinical tutor. Osler had written that when he considered all of his lifetime achievements, the one he felt was of most value was teaching medical students. The seed was planted.

I was by then confident of my abilities to teach GP registrars, but medical students were different. Registrars were qualified and experienced doctors who could make independent clinical decisions. Medical students could not work independently and required constant supervision. I would be required to have a student in my practice for eighteen weeks every six months. My role would be to help them to apply the basic science that they had learned in their first two years in medical school to the problems of patients attending the surgery, while also teaching them the basics of consultation management and communication skills. Many of my GP colleagues questioned my sanity at taking on such a role. General practice was difficult enough, they said, without adding another layer of complexity. But I applied for the post and was accepted.

On my first day as a tutor, I opened the door of the practice to a young man in a shirt and tie, looking about as uncertain as I felt. My instruction manual had suggested that for the first couple of weeks the student should sit in with the doctor and observe the consultation, so, after a brief introduction to our staff and a very short tour of the premises, I invited him to sit in the corner of my consulting room and offered him a pen and a notebook to record his observations, with the intention of discussing them later.

The first patient on my list was Julie Murphy, a young mother who attended infrequently and who had a tendency to be anxious. However, when I opened her file, I noticed that she owed €150 in unpaid consultation fees. Damn, I said to myself, I wish I hadn't seen that.

If Bridget had been there, I would have asked her to deal with it, but Bridget had left to work for the HSE and Angela, a good-humoured and highly efficient young woman, had taken her place. Angela was still learning the ropes, so it would not be fair to give her this delicate task on her first week in the job. I would have to deal with it myself.

Unpaid bills interfere with my consulting. It is difficult to concentrate on complaints of a sore throat, abdominal pain or feelings of depression while at the same time trying to figure out why this person had not paid me for services I have already given. It is even more difficult to try to formulate a plan that might involve blood tests, further follow-up consultations and medications, while part of my brain is wondering if the patient actually has the means to pay. In Julie's case, I was pretty sure that she had a medical card, so she should not have had to pay for her consultations. I realised, with a sinking heart, that it must have been revoked by the PCRS, or Primary Care Reimbursement Service, and that she was unaware of that development. This could have been because she had not received notification of the cancellation, or because she had put the notice aside and forgotten to follow it up, as is common in busy households. Sometimes people missed a notification about a medical card because they could not read it, due to poor eyesight or lower than average literacy skills; others had medical cards with expiry dates extending well into the future, but the card was still deemed invalid by the PCRS. I had given up trying to find rational explanations for the workings of the PCRS and resorted to reacting to each incident as it arose, rather than trying to figure out a cause. Once a card was cancelled, it could take a long time to have it restored and many people did not have the means to pay doctors' fees or medicine costs in the meantime. Nonetheless, I could not continue to see people without payment: if I was to be of service to anyone, I needed to run a viable business. Much as I disliked it, I could not ignore this aspect of general practice and if Julie did not have a valid medical card, then she was responsible for the payment.

I grew up in a non-business household. My mother and father were always salaried employees. Prior to retirement, my father had managed the local farmers' co-operative. Long after it stopped being financially viable, he continued to work voluntarily, because he could see the value of the co-op to the community of small farmers around Letterfrack. My mother taught in a primary school and did voluntary community work in her free time. This was the ethos of our house: service to community. Money would follow, if the job was well done.

One summer, my younger brother Gerry and his friend, who were both around twelve years old, set up their own business. They picked mussels from among the rocks at Derryinver, in Ballinakill Bay, and set up a stall outside our house, selling them to passers-by. They made a big timber sign and painted MUSSELS FOR SALE on it in bright red letters. My father encouraged them and even helped them to transport their catch from the shore to the house. As happens in a small place, word got around that there were quality mussels for sale outside Gannons' house. A couple of local hotels placed regular orders and before long, the boys were finding it difficult to keep up with the demand. Their days of playing football in the front yard while waiting for someone to notice their sign were over, as they spent most of their time at the shore, waiting for low tide, when they would work, backs bent, filling their crates.

As the success of the business grew, my mother became uneasy. Surely it was not right for twelve-year-olds to be making money like this when there were fishermen who had to go to sea for days to make ends meet? As luck or misfortune would have it, a rumour started that the Derryinver mussels were contaminated by sewage. There was no truth in this: Gerry and Johnny had done their research and had consulted Bob, my uncle-in-law, an ex-seaman, who had been collecting and eating mussels from that same area for years. Bob was quite confident that there was no risk of contamination. Nevertheless, the rumour was too much for my mother, who would have felt responsible if anyone had fallen ill and who was uncomfortable with a home industry such as this, in a family that had no experience of either the sea or business. The boys reluctantly but dutifully shut the business down and went back to playing football in the yard. But Gerry's interest in business had been sparked and today he runs his own successful sports shop in Clifden.

Unlike Gerry, I did not choose business as a career. I chose service to community, or so I believed. I thought the money would look after itself, but I was wrong. I could not pay staff salaries, professional fees, my mortgage, meet overheads and buy equipment if I did not pay attention to my income. In the early days of the practice, the desire to provide good-quality care, while making sure I was getting adequately reimbursed, was something I struggled with. This was partly due to my upbringing, but also due to the fact that I had had no business training as a GP registrar. The training Liam and I had received in the UK consisted of two years of hospital posts and one year in a GP practice. While we did learn practice organisation alongside clinical and communication skills, there was very little instruction on running a business. This was probably because in the UK, everyone was entitled to free GP care. There was no exchange of money between doctor and patient, no such thing as unpaid consultation fees. Such was my level of disinterest that to this day, I am not clear on the exact method of GP reimbursement in the UK. As far as I was aware, patients appeared to have no problems getting to see a doctor, doctors made a good living and everyone was happy. I was not long back in Ireland when I realised that a whole section of my education had been neglected. I was ill-equipped for Irish general practice, because I did not know how to charge for my services and had no experience of making sure I got paid.

One evening in 1991, not long after returning to Ireland, Liam and I attended a Continuing Medical Education (CME) meeting in Kilkenny. These small-group monthly meetings are still the preferred way for GPs to keep up to date with fast-paced changes in medicine. They are held countrywide and facilitated by an Irish College of General Practice CME tutor. At this time, Liam had just taken up a temporary GP post in the rural town of Thomastown and both he and I were assigned to the Kilkenny group. These were the days when GPs rarely got a full night's sleep and were on call most weekends. Liam and I, young, optimistic and naïve, were full of enthusiasm, looking forward to working independently and experiencing life in Ireland after our four years in exile. Our optimism was either admirable or foolish, considering the fact that the reason we had a practice to work in was that the incumbent GP had taken up a post in Saudi Arabia in order to improve his financial situation. Nevertheless, we were undaunted.

After the official educational meeting was over, everyone drifted towards the bar. Liam mingled easily with the group of young to middle-aged male GPs, as if he was simply reuniting with old college friends. I was not as relaxed. My tendency to be reserved in the company of those I do not know had been strengthened by spending four years in the UK away from my family and well-established friends.

While Liam and the larger group gravitated towards one end of the bar, I found myself beside an older gentleman in a tweed jacket, who stood apart from the crowd, but who despite this, had a friendly, open demeanour. He introduced himself as Dr Devlin and offered to buy me a drink. I accepted, relieved that he was happy to engage in conversation and followed him to a quieter area of the bar. I sat myself on a high stool and we fell into conversation.

I explained that we had just arrived in Co. Kilkenny, having completed three years of GP training in the UK.

'How times have changed,' he replied. 'Most of the GPs of my vintage did a few years in hospital and then put up their plate. A bit more training might have been good alright.'

'Oh, I don't know,' I said. 'Most of the training is on the job. I know we both still have a lot to learn.'

Dr Devlin laughed. 'Lots that you won't find on any GP-training scheme.'

He continued to question me on the rationale of coming back to Ireland when everyone else our age was heading off to America on the Morrison visas, the lottery which had provided visas to eligible Irish emigrants in the early 1990s. I realised that ours was not a rational decision, more an emotional one. Most of the class of 1986, the year that Liam and I qualified, had gone to the UK after completing an internship year and we did not yet know of anyone who had returned. But Ireland was our home and we would never be happy if we did not try to build a life here. I borrowed a reply from an engineer friend, also an Irish graduate who had emigrated to the UK and who was planning to return as soon as possible. 'Surely we will find one job in the whole of the country. It's not as if we are trying to set up an industry or anything.'

The conversation flowed and before long I had forgotten the others, forgotten that I was new to the area, that I was the only woman at the meeting, recovered something of the old me, who connected with Irish wit and humour and who disregarded age and gender.

Eventually, the conversation came around to money. 'If you don't ask for it, you won't get it and if you think someone is trying to pull a fast one, you're probably right,' Dr Devlin said. 'And if that is the case, don't let them out of your sight until they have handed it over.' This last sentence was uttered with the same degree of gravity that I had once heard a consultant anaesthetist use to instruct a junior doctor not to insert a tracheal tube until the patient was actually asleep. 'I'm telling you this now,' he went on, 'but I wasn't always so wise myself.' He nodded to the barman to bring us another drink. I rummaged in my bag for my purse, but he motioned me to put it away. I didn't feel I could insist.

'I'd say I was a bit older than yourself when I had my first lesson in extracting money,' he said, laughing. 'I haven't told this story in a while, but you might find it instructive, seeing as we're all here for an educational meeting.' He took a sip of his Guinness, wiped a layer of froth off his upper lip, set his pint on the counter and went on. 'I wasn't long in practice here in Kilkenny when a certain businessman, who had obviously sniffed out my lack of prowess in financial matters, succeeded in owing me a lot of money. He was a shopkeeper here in town, dead now, God rest him. He called me out to see his son after surgery one day. The son, a young fellow of about thirteen, was in bed with a high temperature, pain all over, swollen joints in his hands and feet and a rash.'

'Rheumatic fever,' I said, unable to help myself, as if it was a medical quiz.

'The very thing,' Dr Devlin replied. 'I arranged an ambulance for him to go to hospital, where he was treated with antibiotics and recovered well. The father was keen that I keep an eye on him. He knew you could get heart damage from rheumatic fever and thought that every cough or sniffle needed to be checked. I could understand that, of course.

'It was a bit of a chore going to visit him at home after surgery and eventually I suggested that he was probably well enough to come in to me, but the parents were busy in the shop and they were worried that he might pick up an infection in the surgery, so I lost that battle. Eventually, I sent him to a heart specialist in Dublin, who checked him from head to toe and told them he had no heart problems, but at this stage the whole family treated him as an invalid.'

'The poor young fellow,' I said. 'It can't have been easy for him to make sense of all that medical attention. How did you manage him after that?'

Dr Devlin took another sip of his pint and went on. 'I continued to go to the house whenever they called, but I was getting a bit uneasy as the bill was getting bigger and bigger and there was no sign of anyone paying it. In the beginning, I didn't like to mention it. They were worried and upset about him being sick and I thought it might be a bit indelicate to talk about money. But when, after weeks and months of me visiting the house, there was still no mention of money, I had a quiet word with the father, saying that it was adding up and trying to be as diplomatic as possible, asked him how he would like to pay, cash or cheque. He apologised profusely and said he would send the wife in with the chequebook without delay.

'A couple of weeks passed and there was no sign of her and I had to mention it again. They continued to call me to the house, even though the young lad was now back at school and fully recovered. There was never a mention of payment and always some excuse as to why he couldn't pay that day, if I mentioned it. I eventually realised that he had no intention of paying at all.'

I found it hard to believe that someone would keep calling a doctor and not pay them, especially someone who, in all likelihood, was not short of money. I also found it hard to believe that a doctor would keep going to a house when it was obvious that they didn't want to pay him. I said this to Dr Devlin.

'Well, I didn't really want to refuse. I was always afraid not to go out when called, in case there was something seriously wrong. I felt a bit trapped as, by all accounts, the father was a reasonable man and I had never heard anyone say a bad word about him. Of, course, I didn't really have anyone I could ask about him, without disclosing that I was seeing his son and that he wasn't paying me. I was afraid that this would be a breach of confidentiality.'

I could understand that. Breach of confidentiality could lead to a Medical Council investigation and no doctor wanted to bring that on themselves.

Dr Devlin explained that he was beginning to get annoyed by the man's audacity and knew he had to do something about it. After a long slug of his pint of Guinness, he continued in the even, relaxed manner of a man who, I imagined, would be difficult to provoke. 'Late enough one evening, I wandered in to the shop. It was a draper's that sold good-quality suits and jackets. I decided I could do with a new suit. The father spotted me as I walked in and had great welcome for me. I tried on a few suits, twisting and turning in front of the mirror, him letting me know that whatever I fancied could be let out, taken in, lengthened or shortened – nothing was too much trouble.

'I settled on one and was just taking it off when out he came with a matching shirt and tie. I wasn't really planning on buying that much, but he convinced me. He insisted that it was a pity to spend that much on a suit and not show it off properly, for want of a new shirt and tie. He offered to let me take them home and show them to the wife and if she didn't like them, I could bring them back. I reluctantly agreed. Next, I saw him coming with a pair of shoes, a beautiful pair of tan Winstanleys. He knew his job, this man. He was a top-class salesman. I said I was OK for shoes, but he would not be dissuaded. I tried them on and he told me to take them away with me and bring them back if I decided I didn't like them. I could tell he was delighted with himself and, while he was packing them up, we chatted away about the hurling, the state of the economy and how business was slow.

'Eventually, he stopped talking and went into the back office to calculate the damage. There was no till or calculators in those days, but he had it all totted up fairly fast. It came to a fair bit. He praised me on my choice of suit, saying that it would be well worth the money, as I should get years of wear out of it. Then he made a bit of a deal about crossing off the shirt and giving me that for free, seeing as how I had spent so much.'

'I presume you were going to negotiate a sizeable discount,' I said, laughing. 'You had certainly earned it.'

Dr Devlin raised his eyebrows and chuckled to himself before continuing. 'I bent down to pick up the bags, while he hovered over me, waiting for me to produce my wallet or chequebook. I'll never forget the look on his face when he realised that I had no intention of paying. I can still see his expression. Pure disbelief and shock. His colour even changed to a slight purple. For once, he had no words. I could tell the thought had never crossed his mind and if he could have grabbed the bags back off me, he would have, but I had a tight hold on them and by then was already half-way out the door.' Dr Devlin laughed.

I could tell it was not just a tall tale by the way he still enjoyed the memory. 'So, you just walked out without paying,' I said.

'You bet your life I did,' he said. 'Sure, didn't he owe me that much and more, and he'd had loads of chances to pay. You bet your life I didn't pay. And I didn't bring any of them back either.'

'So that was it, you just took the bags and left?'

'Well, no, not exactly. I told him that Margaret, my wife, had the chequebook gone with her to Dublin, but she would be in some day to sort it out. But sure we both knew that would never happen.'

'So, what happened the next time he called you out to see his son?' I asked.

'I never got another call,' Dr Devlin replied. 'And I was very glad I didn't. That, my girl, is the sort of business you can do without.'

This was a story I had re-told many times, but it wasn't going to help me in any way to deal with Julie's unpaid consultations

I opened the door and called Julie from the waiting room. She rushed in past me with her usual sense of urgency, which I had grown accustomed to, but had learned to ignore. She nodded a brief hello to the medical student, who had stood up to greet her, as if it was nothing out of the ordinary to have someone sitting in the corner while she consulted me and before any of us had a chance to sit down, she started talking. I presumed that Angela had asked her to sign the consent form, stating that she did not mind the student remaining in the room and would have liked to have asked her this myself, just to be sure, but she did not give me a chance.

'It's just something very small, doctor,' she said. 'I won't keep you a minute. I can see how busy you are.'

My intention to put my cards clearly on the table, to clarify the unpaid bills, didn't stand a chance. We were right in the scene of the action with no clear rules of engagement. I had no choice but to shelve my own agenda and let her tell me what was on her mind.

Julie continued speaking, her sentences tumbling out, one on top of the other, unrestrained and effusive. The ratio of signal to noise made it difficult to decipher her core problem, which eventually began to emerge as a pain in her abdomen that went around to her back and down her leg. This was a pretty routine problem for a GP, but one that required careful history-taking, examination, investigation and possible referral. Certainly not an issue that would only 'keep me a minute'.

I let her speak until she began to repeat herself and then interrupted her. 'OK, let me just summarise. I think what you are saying is … ' I started to repeat what I had heard in my own words. My intention was to make sure that I had understood exactly what she was worried about.

I was half-way through the next sentence when she cut in again, saying, 'Yes, that's right and then it went round to my back and ...'

I remained silent and let her go on for a couple of seconds. When she eventually took a breath, I grabbed the chance to interject. 'I did hear that, Julie, but can you just let me say it back to you, so that you can be sure I understand? I will then go on to do an examination and we can make a plan.'

In consulting terms, this is called 'signposting', explicitly pointing out how the consultation will proceed, so that the patient knows how the doctor is planning to manage the problem. GP consultations need a structure if they are to be effective. This cannot be rigid, considering the vast array of problems that people present with, but there are some useful techniques that work well to prevent consultations going round and round in circles, where the patient keeps saying the same thing over and over, because they think the doctor has not heard or does not understand their meaning. Or consultations where the doctor gets lost, their mind wandering back to the previous patient, to the house call that needs to be organised, or the logistics of getting out in time for a parent–teacher meeting. Signposting is one of these techniques.

Effective consultations, ones that end with both doctor and patient reaching a shared understanding and a clear management plan, rarely happen by chance. What appears to the casual observer a straightforward interchange between a patient presenting their problem and a doctor offering their solution, takes skill and practice and, even now, I often get it wrong. I am always actively trying to improve my consultations, but on that occasion, knowing that I was being observed by a medical student, I was even more conscious of this.

My consultation skills guru in those days was an English GP named Roger Neighbour. My bible was a book written by him, first published in 1987, called *The Inner Consultation: how to develop an effective and intuitive consulting style.* This book emphasised the importance of doctors developing awareness of their own personalities and emotions alongside clinical competence. As someone who read psychology in my free time and had toyed with the idea of becoming a psychiatrist, I loved the way in which this book encouraged me, as a medical doctor, to continuously monitor the unconscious forces that were at work in my personal and professional life. It also validated my increasing conviction that my behaviour during a consultation was just as important as that of the patient.

In addition to its erudite and multi-layered content, the book provided a checklist of five easy-to-remember, deceptively simple actions that could keep any consultation on track. Describing it as a journey for doctor and patient, these five actions were presented as checkpoints that doctors could try to reach, stopping there a while to see if both doctor and patient were going in the same direction, at the same speed. The actions were connecting, summarising, handing over, safety-netting and housekeeping. Whenever I felt that either I or the patient was off track during a consultation, I would silently assess whether we had reached any of these checkpoints and gently guide the patient to that place where we could slow down and plan the rest of the journey. This could be done unobtrusively, when I was not tired or stressed or rushed. I had read *The Inner Consultation* so often that on some days I felt the presence of Roger Neighbour on my shoulder, gently nudging me in one direction or another.

Many years previously, my friend Myriam and I had travelled to Edinburgh to sit the oral part of the GP membership examination. This is an examination that allows qualified GPs to attain membership of the Royal College of General Practitioners. At the time, it was desirable, but not compulsory, for all newly qualified GPs to have passed. It was to be my second time sitting this examination, having failed the oral section the first time.

Myriam took advantage of my prior experience the night before the exam, in our shared hotel room, and quizzed me on what she was likely to be asked.

'They often ask if you have read anything interesting that helps your consulting,' I replied.

Myriam thought for a minute. 'I haven't really read anything about consulting,' she said. 'I've been too busy working.' It was 1991 and Myriam was in her final year of GP training in Galway while I had just finished my training in the UK. 'What about you?' she asked. 'Have you read anything you can tell me about?'

I produced my copy of the *The Inner Consultation* and handed it over to her, explaining that I dipped in and out of it when I got a chance and that it had helped me to manage my consulting.

She flicked through it and frowned. 'Not a chance I will read that before morning,' she said, looking through the book with a resigned air. She stopped at a page and held it out to me, pointing out the word PITSTOP standing alone at the end of a paragraph. 'Why is PITSTOP printed in bold like that at the end of some of the paragraphs?' she asked.

I explained that PITSTOP indicated that you should stop reading, put the book down and reflect on what you had just read. Even if you wanted to continue, you would get more benefit from the book if you actually stopped reading at that point.

'Interesting,' she said, letting the book fall on to the bed. 'I'll just have to hope they don't ask me about books I have read.'

The following day we turned up for the exam and were assigned to two different sets of examiners. As the interview was coming to a close, one of the three men on Myriam's examination panel said he would like to ask her one last question. Had she read anything interesting recently that she found useful for her consultations and if she had, how was it useful? Without hesitation, Myriam flashed a ready smile at her examiners and declared that the most useful book she had ever read on the consultation, dangerously implying that she had read more than one, was *The Inner Consultation* by Roger Neighbour. Before she could be interrupted, she went on to explain how the idea of having PITSTOPS in the book had benefited her enormously in absorbing the contents and applying them to her own consultations. They were such a good idea that she was trying to impose this discipline on herself when reading other books.

They smiled back, thanked her for attending and wished her well in her career.

As we packed up our bags for home, Myriam retrieved the book from where it had lain since the night before. As she handed it to me, she suddenly stopped and her face went a little pale. 'Lucia,' she said, pointing to the picture of a smiling, slightly balding man on the back of the book, 'Please don't tell me that that is Roger Neighbour?'

I peered at the photograph. 'Well, of course it is,' I said. 'Who else would it be?'

'He was one of my examiners,' she said slowly. 'Oh, my God. There I was, going on about his book and he was sitting in front of me and I didn't even recognise him.'

'Are you sure?' I asked, a little bit envious that she had got him and I hadn't. I would at least have recognised him *and* I had read the book.

'Absolutely,' she replied. 'He was a little older, but it was definitely him.'

We were both looking at the picture. Myriam began to read the last line of the author biography. 'Roger Neighbour ... a fellow of the Royal College of General Practitioners, he is currently a member of its panel of examiners.'

'I'm sure he was suitably charmed,' I said, trying to put her at ease. I did not know anyone, male or female, who would not be charmed by this intelligent, attractive, engaging, stylishly dressed young woman, with her genuine smile and air of complete confidence.

I was right. She passed with flying colours. I was lucky to scrape through.

Now, I knew I had to slow Julie down, to get her to stop rushing through her problems, but before I had a chance to go on, Julie was speaking again. 'Right, Doctor,' she said, placing her bag on the floor and jumping up, already making her way to the couch.

'No, Julie, sit for a minute, while I recap on what you just told me and clarify a few other important things with you.' I finally managed to summarise her complaint and invited her to get up on the couch so that I could do an examination. This phase of the consultation was usually a time of quiet. A time when I could gather my thoughts and consider what the next step was. The familiar, ritualistic process of examining patients calmed me, brought me back to the present, blocked out intruding thoughts and reminded me of my most important tasks; history-taking, examination, diagnosis and management. Even nowadays, when every part of the body can be visualised on a machine; when an MRI is a household term, even if its limitations are poorly understood; when the CT scan has been superseded by the even more powerful PET scan as the ultimate tool for detecting damaged organs and aberrant cells, a careful physical examination is the most important initial procedure and should not be omitted.

I let Julie settle on the couch, lowering the headrest and adjusting the pillow under her head to help her get comfortable. I picked up her hand and was just about to take her pulse when she started talking again.

'Oh, before I forget it, Doctor, I just wanted to ask you about my daughter. She is not well. I didn't bring her in, because she is not that bad, really, and I didn't want to take up too much of your time. She went to school today, but I am afraid she will get worse and I wonder if I could get her an antibiotic?'

I didn't reply. I carried on examining her pulse as if I had not heard her speak. I was still processing her initial complaint. I didn't know what the pain in her abdomen that went around to her back and down her leg was. The pain that woke her at night and put her off her daily walks, that meant she had to sit down to do her ironing. The pain that she thought might be ovarian cancer, because her aunt had had ovarian cancer in her forties. Surely, this was the main reason she was in. This was what I needed to concentrate on, but she was handing me more balls to juggle and despite being an adept multitasker, I was as likely to drop one as anyone else.

'I'll deal with you first,' I said, when I had finished checking her pulse. 'I think we have enough to be getting on with here for the moment.' I had no intention of getting back to talk about her daughter. I had no intention of giving an antibiotic for a child who was not even present.

'Oh sorry, Doctor,' she replied. 'I just didn't want to take up another appointment. I know how busy you are.' She had sensed my annoyance. She smiled as she said this and I knew she was genuine.

'I will always have an appointment for a sick child,' I said. 'If you are worried, it's best to bring her in.'

I was training myself to stop trying to do too much in each consultation. Multitasking might work for making the dinner and cleaning the house, but it was not a good idea in the surgery. Forgetting to light the gas under the green beans because I had decided to fold the laundry was not the same as forgetting to send a letter for a potential malignant melanoma because I had allowed myself to get distracted talking about a sore toe, or a letter for the council. Now that I was established in practice, I was less worried that people might think I was being contrary when I declined to deal with multiple problems and more concerned with practising good, safe medicine and protecting myself from feeling overwhelmed. I realised I was actually becoming much more adept at saying 'no'.

I completed the examination in silence and, when I was finished, indicated that she should sit back down in the chair. When she was settled and I had her attention, I began to explain my plan. This was the 'handing-over' checkpoint, where I shared my plan with the patient and allowed her to make adjustments. It was at this point that I needed Julie to commit to whatever course of action we chose to take. 'So, this is what I think ... '

She interrupted me again. 'It's nothing serious is it, Doctor?'

'No, I don't think so,' I replied. 'I haven't felt anything in your abdomen that should not be there.'

'Oh, good,' she replied. 'But what is it then, Doctor?'

'Well, if you just let me explain,' I said. 'I was going to say that, even though I do not think there is anything serious wrong, I do think you need a couple more investigations.'

She started to cry. 'You think it is cancer, Doctor,' she said. 'Like my aunt. This is exactly what happened to her.'

I sat back and moved the tissue box within her reach so she could blow her nose and dry the tears that had started to drop from her cheek on to her lap. 'No,' I said. 'I definitely do not think you have cancer.'

I suddenly remembered the three unpaid consultations and while giving her a chance to recover her equilibrium, glanced at the 'private health insurance' item on her file. It was blank. I wondered again about her financial situation. She needed an abdominal ultrasound at minimum, but she would have to pay for this if she wanted it any sooner than in six months' time. I could refer her to a clinic, but which one? Without a scan it was a random choice between gynaecology, renal and gastroenterology and if I got it wrong, she would wait for six months at least to be assessed and then be sent back to me to be referred for another scan. If I only had her health needs to consider, it would have been easy, but every time I made a plan for a patient such as this, I also had to consider their financial situation. The two were inseparable. I really wished this lady still had her medical card. At least then she would be saved the cost of GP consultations and might manage to pay for a private ultrasound. The prospect of addressing the three unpaid consultations was getting more remote.

Julie had dried her tears and was sitting forward in her chair, ready to listen. I asked her if she had medical insurance, but she shook her head. I asked her if she would consider a private ultrasound. She responded that it would be a struggle to pay for it.

I decided to broach the subject of her finances in general directly. 'Julie,' I asked her. 'Are you struggling financially at the moment and is that a source of stress for you?' Stress from any source can augment physical symptoms and steal a person's reserves, leading to all sorts of imagined illnesses. The ease with which she had started to cry when I'd mentioned further tests was evidence of her fragility.

She answered that things were no worse than usual and asked me why I thought that might be a factor.

'Well, it's just that to get further tests privately will be expensive and I just noticed before you came in that the last three consultations here were unpaid.'

Julie looked at me in surprise. 'Three unpaid consultations?' she said. 'But that's impossible. I have a medical card. You know that. I have always had a medical card.' She automatically picked up the handbag she had left beside her chair and started to rummage in it, eventually pulling out a wallet and, finally, her medical card. She handed it over to me and sure enough it was still in date, the expiry date not for another eighteen months. Whatever the reason, it was Angela who had found out that the card had been cancelled, that we had not been paid for Julie's recent consultations and would not be paid for this one. I had no energy left to explain this to Julie, so I told her to talk to Angela on the way out and she would tell her what she needed to do to get her card restored.

After veering off track into murky financial waters, I shifted gear and resumed my medical journey with Julie, who decided to go for a private ultrasound. I provided her with a referral letter and we progressed to the fourth checkpoint, safety-netting. This involved giving instructions to her to come back if things got worse, if any new symptoms appeared, or if she had any trouble getting an appointment. Finally, she left, thanking me and reassuring me that she understood our plan and would follow it.

As I closed the door, I progressed to the fifth and final checkpoint, housekeeping. I sat for a minute before making my notes and acknowledged to myself that even though, on the surface, there was nothing complicated about Julie's medical problems and that I was well within my comfort zone medically, the consultation had been difficult and multi-layered and that I was tired and drained.

I turned to the medical student, who had been sitting quietly in the corner, ostensibly observing everything. 'Well, any observations on all that?' I asked, considering this an appropriate open-ended question that would bring forth an unbiased reply.

'Not really,' he answered. 'Pretty straightforward. Nothing too complicated.' He glanced quickly at the notepad I had given him, as if wanting to be reminded of some important insight or observation that he had noted earlier. I was almost certain that it was blank.

'You're right,' I replied with a smile. 'Nothing to it, really. About as straightforward as you will get.'

Later that evening, my friend Judith and I were walking in the bog. It was early autumn and the brambles were heavy with blackberries, the unharvested bog awash with a multitude of purple, pink and lilac, heather, loosestrife and bartsia. As we circled the lake for the last time, the sun was beginning to go down. Judith's dog Tao, a husky who loved to run free on these walks, stopped on the little jetty looking, Narcissus-like, at his reflection in the water. We both joined him, sitting on the sides of the jetty, looking out to the island on the lake, the water calm and still. Beside us the pale, delicate water lilies were in full bloom. Out of the almost motionless reeds a family of ducks emerged, gliding smoothly over the surface, a perfect V-shaped fan of water extending out behind each one.

'They are so graceful,' Judith said. 'And they make it look so effortless. It's hard to believe that they are paddling away like mad under the water.'

'I can well believe it,' I replied, before turning for home.

CHAPTER TWELVE

SPREAD A LITTLE HAPPINESS

I t was the shortest day of the year. The trees stood stark and bare against the grey sky, the few copper and brown leaves that still clung to their branches a sad reminder of sunnier times. As if to add to the dreariness the rain that morning was relentless. I flicked on the switch to the Christmas tree lights in the waiting room as I passed by. The place was already busy and it appeared that nobody had noticed this omission. My consulting room, usually bright and sunny, was dark and uninviting. I took off my new rain jacket and hung it on the coat rail in my room, noting the little puddles of water that formed on the floor underneath it. I also noticed, with annoyance, that the bottom of my skirt and my tights were wet, even though I had only travelled the short path from the house to the surgery. I pressed the button to turn on the computer, moved a pile of papers off my work space and sat down. There was no point hoping that the surgery would be quiet. It was always busier in wet weather and especially just before Christmas. Everybody wanted to be well for Christmas and everybody wanted to know what day we would close and what day we would re-open. To make matters worse, everyone who came in would complain about the weather. And it would be impossible to examine anyone, as they would be muffled up in layers of clothes that would take for ever to peel off. The waiting room floor would be covered in little puddles of water, just like the ones under my coat. The air would be heavy with moisture, the coatstand in the waiting room decorated with forgotten, unloved hats, scarves and umbrellas at the end of the morning.

All these negative thoughts were going through my head as I waited to get into my HealthOne computer program and see what was in store for me that morning. HealthOne is a program designed by GPs to help with all our daily tasks, such as setting up appointments, recording medical histories, referring to secondary care, auditing our practice and lots of other clever functions that I have yet to master. I often wonder how I ever managed to accomplish anything before it became available. Now, as the familiar appointment screen came into view, I noticed that my first patient was Monica, a lady in her early seventies, who was always in a good mood and who never left the surgery without having something positive to say. Today will test her, I thought. Nobody could possibly be in a good mood today.

I had been grumpy all morning and everything that had happened since I had set foot out of bed transpired to keep me that way. As I had woken Ailshe and Liam Jnr for school, it had been difficult to disguise my irritability. Liam Jnr had subsequently forgotten his lunch, meaning I would have to drive the ten miles into Thurles to give it to him when I had finished surgery, otherwise he would never survive the day. Caredoc, the out-of-hours co-operative, had called at eight o'clock that morning to say a patient had died over the weekend and Liam had gone out early to visit the family. There would be no time for that later in the day. I had barely acknowledged the poor family's grief. My mind had only registered the fact that I would have to be the one to take Dax, our new Labrador, a would-be guide dog who had defied his destiny by being too distractable, for his morning walk, in the pouring rain.

Despite the fact that I had been nurturing all these reasons to be negative, I couldn't help but feel a slight change of perspective as I looked again at Monica's name. If I had to see anyone, Monica was a good antidote to grumpiness. It could just happen that her cheerfulness would rub off on me rather than my negativity transfer to her. There was no doubt that work was good for me: there in my consulting seat, getting ready to start my day, I felt myself step outside my negative thoughts and take on the responsibility of not transferring my mood to others. This did not happen so easily at home, but at work, along with being clinically competent, there was the need to be cheerful and positive for the sake of the patients.

A GP friend had scoffed at me when I tried to explain this to her one day. 'You take your responsibilities far too seriously, Lucia,' she had laughed. 'You are not responsible for anyone's mood except your own. We are not robots who can be programmed to be positive. You feel what you feel and even if you try to hide it, people see through it anyway.'

I was not convinced. I knew that sometimes I could be so attuned to the mental state of another that I subconsciously adopted this state. This was advantageous if they were feeling good, but was not so great if they were feeling bad. And if that was the case for me then it was probably also the case for others. I also believed that it was possible to decide to be positive rather than negative and thereby alter negative feelings. Looking again at the screen, I noticed that my appointments were not full, which meant I was unlikely to have extras and would get out early enough to go to Thurles with the forgotten lunch. I was already halfway to cheerful as I called Monica in and even managed a smile as I held the door open for her.

'Good morning, Doctor Gannon,' Monica said, with her usual cheerfulness. 'Aren't you great to be in and ready for action so early, on such a bad day.'

I am indeed, I thought, feeling good about myself for the first time that morning. 'Well, in fairness, I didn't have far to travel,' I said. 'It's one good thing about living so close to my work. I can't complain about the traffic or the weather.'

I was standing beside her waiting to take her coat, so that I could hang it up alongside my own. I liked to take the patient's jacket or coat and hang it up while they settled themselves in the chair. It was a way of welcoming people to my space, as I would do if they came to my home. A way of indicating that I would like them to be comfortable and relaxed. At a deeper level, this shedding of the outer layer was intended as an invitation to connect, to expose something of their inner selves, if that is what they needed to do. There were those who never removed their coats or jackets and that was their right. That was their comfort level and I respected that. But there was another reason I liked to be in charge of the coats and jackets: some people were inclined to overstay their welcome and when this happened, I would take that same coat or jacket off the hook, stand beside the patient and hold it out to help them put it back on. There could be no mistaking my gesture. As far as I was concerned, business had been completed.

Monica was struggling out of her wet and dripping beige raincoat while trying to avoid leaving an equally wet and glistening plastic headscarf on my desk. I was about to help her when I remembered that she was one of the few who would never allow me to do this for her. She turned her back on me, clasping the dripping garments to her and made her way to the row of hooks on the wall behind my chair. 'Now, Doctor Gannon,' she said. 'I've told you before. You have enough to do without hanging up coats for the likes of me. I don't expect anyone to wait on me like that. Sit down there now. I'll be with you in a minute.'

I did as I was told. I sat into my chair and felt the tension leave my shoulders. My breathing slowed and deepened, my jaw and gaze softened. My consulting room, dark and uninviting a short time before, was gradually filling with warmth and light. The rain still spattered against the window and I heard the wind picking up outside, but this only heightened my sense of comfort and privilege. The tangled, frazzled, edgy feelings I had had earlier in the morning loosened their grip and were soon forgotten. I was suddenly feeling very fortunate. Fortunate to have an indoor occupation. Fortunate to be in good health, to have three healthy children, even if they were a bit forgetful at times, and fortunate to have a husband who always did the early-morning and late-night calls.

Monica smoothed down her skirt and came to sit opposite me. It struck me that she was probably oblivious to the positive influence she had on me that morning and, through me, on all the others I would encounter that day. I had spent years learning and practising communication skills in order to connect and heal and help people along difficult paths. Monica seemed to have this innate ability without any training. She emanated genuine warmth and caring and spread this among those she met. She did not distinguish between those who needed care and those, like me, who were expected to provide it. She gave equally to everyone. As the consultation unfolded, my disgruntled air dissipated and through the window, I noticed that the sun had now risen and that the day was considerably brighter.

Monica rose to leave, making her way to the coat hooks. There was no danger of her overstaying her welcome. 'Thank you so much, Doctor,' she said. It's always good to see you.'

'I think I benefited a lot more from seeing you today than you did from me,' I laughed, as I handed her a six-month script. 'I think I got out of the wrong side of the bed this morning and was in danger of nursing my grievances all day, until I saw you.'

'You have a hard job, but I'm glad you do it, and I hope you know that. I don't know what we would do without yourself and Doctor Liam. Now, I'd better not delay you any longer. You have a lot of people out there who are a lot sicker than me.'

I held the door open and noticed that she touched me lightly on the shoulder, as she left. 'Have a lovely Christmas and I'll see you in six months,' she said.

After she left, I thought about how lucky she was to have been born with such a positive and grateful disposition. I had been studying the subject of happiness, as part of a masters degree in applied positive psychology. Positive psychology was a relatively new discipline that had come to my attention through a book called *Authentic Happiness* by Martin Seligman, the study of what keeps well people well, which made a welcome change from thinking about illness and disease. I had read that there is evidence that everyone is born with a particular happiness set-point. I suspected Monica's was high, but I also guessed that she worked at maintaining it. Happiness, I was discovering, was tightly bound to gratitude and appreciation and it was worth pursuing, not as advocated by the many popular psychology books, which implied that telling yourself you were happy would make it so. It was not as simple as that. Real happiness involved actively developing a genuine appreciation of life and its treasures. Happiness was itself a virtue which could be used to spread further happiness. Doing good helped people feel good, but feeling good helped people do good, and so it was possible to create an upward spiral of wellbeing for ourselves, which then helped us to connect with others and caused them to also feel well. Just as a stone dropped into water could change the whole pond, so, too, could an act of kindness or an expression of gratitude cause a ripple effect of goodwill, spreading outwards with immeasurable effects. Monica simply embodied what I had read.

Richard Bach, author of *Jonathan Livingston Seagull,* once wrote: 'We teach best what we most need to learn.' It might have been for this reason that I frequently found myself preparing educational workshops in my role as assistant programme director with the South-East GP training scheme, on topics that I wanted to understand more deeply, topics that had not been taught in college or in my GP training, but knowledge of which made my work easier and more enjoyable. One Wednesday afternoon, not long after this consultation with Monica, I decided to present the topic of positive emotion and wellbeing and bring to the group all the questions I had and all the theories and evidence I had read. The registrars in my group had already completed their hospital training and were all working in GP practices, with a GP trainer. They would have to complete a further year in a different GP practice, pass the membership exam for the Irish College of General Practitioners, get signed off on a women's health module and a contraception certificate, complete an immediate-care course, a research or audit project and submit assessments from all their training posts, before they could be regarded as fully fledged competent GPs. The shift from hospital to GP was challenging. While they could ask their GP trainer for advice and guidance at any time, they were expected, throughout these years, to make independent, autonomous decisions, to manage acute emergencies, to treat people with multiple diseases, to prescribe safely and cost-effectively and to use secondary care services appropriately.

The registrars met on Wednesdays for their educational meetings. sessions which were derisively labelled 'Play School' by some of the hospital doctors, who had no idea what sort of learning took place during the meetings and who were probably a little envious of the protected time that these doctors were allocated for group learning. But these trainee GPs, once qualified, could potentially end up working alone – unlike hospital doctors – with no team, no supervision, no one to confer with. To spend an afternoon exploring 'positive emotion' would be considered by some a waste of time and effort, but as well as clinical knowledge and practical skills I knew that these new doctors would need to be competent in managing their emotions, in dealing with uncertainty, living with the consequences of their decisions and with accepting their impotence to alter the course of some people's lives. These processes can be much more difficult than managing blood pressure, providing antenatal care or operating on an appendix. These small-group sessions provided a safe place where doctors could share their experiences, realise that the things they found challenging were the same for all, and could develop self-awareness and enhanced confidence in their own abilities to meet and deal with the challenges they encountered.

On that particular afternoon, I had started the session with my usual question. 'So, who knows what we will be doing today?' I had posted the agenda for the meeting on Moodle, the online interactive platform used by all the registrars and educators to keep abreast of what was going on, but I wouldn't have been surprised if nobody had got around to reading it.

I got the usual response: two of the twelve hands went up. Others pulled apologetic faces, raised their eyebrows, or drew in their breath, before emitting quiet 'sorry' sounds and offering me half-smiles, to let me know that no offence or disrespect was intended. They were simply busy and had, as I had suspected, not got around to it. I was used to this and it didn't bother me. In fact, I was sometimes glad when registrars came to these sessions with no knowledge of the content, no preconceived ideas, no prepared responses to the questions posed. These were often the liveliest, most spontaneous and most enjoyable sessions.

Now I began tentatively, expecting resistance, scepticism and even withdrawal. 'My aim for this session is to discuss positive emotion,' I said, 'What it is, how we experience it, how we can experience more of it and why this is a good thing.'

The twelve faces remained expressionless. I imagined I heard a groan. I became aware of a wall, possibly not yet impenetrable, being built in their heads. For these scientifically minded young professionals, talking about wishy-washy subjects like 'feelings' or 'positivity' was akin to dabbling in the occult. I did not have much of a window, so I explained that the session was based on the scientific research of Dr Rick Hanson, a neuroscientist and psychologist, and Dr Barbara Fredrickson, a clinical psychologist. Both had spent their professional lives researching the physiological and behavioural effects of emotions. Even though none of the group had heard of either of these people, I sensed we were back on familiar territory and the mood of the group shifted again to one of guarded receptivity and mild curiosity. A neuroscientist and a clinical psychologist were worthy of some attention.

Throughout the session we discussed the idea of a 'happiness set-point,' which implies that regardless of what happens in our lives, we all revert to a pre-determined level of wellbeing, once the events are over. We explored the concept of a 'negativity bias,' which means that we are more inclined to dwell on negative than positive events. We redefined for ourselves the term 'positive emotion', which is commonly thought to mean indefinable happiness, but can actually be broken down into emotions such as gratitude, compassion, love or awe. We discussed Barbara Fredrickson's 'broaden and build' theory, which shows that when we experience any positive emotion, it broadens our thinking, improves our problem-solving abilities and helps us to build relationships through increasing our feelings of connection with others. As the session progressed, I became aware of an enhanced feeling of connection within the group, a heightened level of interest in how this could be applied to themselves and an eagerness to try the techniques suggested to increase positive emotion in both their personal and professional lives. All too soon it was over.

As we were getting ready to leave, Marie, a quiet and thoughtful young woman in her mid-twenties, announced that she had some good news to share. She had just got engaged. The group congratulated her, but also admonished her for not announcing this sooner. She responded to this gentle chastisement by saying that she didn't think people would be that interested and that they would think that she was gloating, or that perhaps if someone was not quite as content with their life as she was, her news would make them feel worse.

As I drove home, I thought about Marie and her reluctance to share her good fortune. I could understand it: I had often made my life appear small so as to allow others to appear bigger. I had often hidden the good and the positive and shared the negative. As Dr Rick Hanson explained, our brains are like 'Teflon for the positive' and 'Velcro for the negative'. It's as if positive experiences do not stick with us for long, while negative ones cling to us, long after they have outlived their usefulness.

Doctors are trained to always scan and search for the negative, to be ready for the worst-case scenario. To be more of an Eeyore than a Pollyanna, or what Edward de Bono described as 'black-hat thinkers', looking for flaws and pitfalls and things that can go wrong. Doctors, as a group with a higher than average suicide rate, could benefit more than most from re-orienting to the positive.

Feeling good makes us reach out to others. Feeling bad makes us withdraw into ourselves. Because we are in the business of caring for others, it is important that we feel good ourselves. Doctors are much more than the prescriptions they write or the medicines they administer, just as teachers are much more than the subjects they teach. As doctors, we can add value to everything we do, if we are happy as we do it. I am convinced that there is nothing wrong with being a little more Pollyanna and a little less Eeyore.

CHAPTER THIRTEEN

A BROKEN PROMISE

I followed the last patient to the door, holding it open as she went out into the dimly lit car park. 'Be careful on the road,' I said, 'it looks frosty.'

It was the end of my day, but as I came back into the waiting room, Angela, the practice secretary, was crouching down behind the counter, coat already on, rooting amidst the stacks of paper and envelopes on the shelves. Beside her, the printer spewed out an A4 document that looked suspiciously like the template letter I usually took with me on a house call, in case a patient needed to be referred to hospital.

She heard me close and lock the door and got to her feet. 'Sorry,' she said, apologising for something that I was sure was not her fault. 'I'm afraid there is an urgent callout to Miss Durkin. It came in just before I switched over the phone to the answering machine and they asked especially for you.' She was concentrating on fitting the document from the printer into the envelope that she had retrieved from the shelf, while avoiding eye contact, well aware that I would not greet this news with enthusiasm.

'What's the problem?' I asked, unable to conceal my irritation. It was annoying when house calls came in late, just when I thought I was finished for the day and was looking forward to getting home. And I was long enough in the job to know that urgent did not always mean urgent.

'It was her neighbour who called,' Angela replied. 'She thinks Miss Durkin fell last night and that she has been lying on the floor until now.' She placed the envelope and document in the emergency doctor's bag. 'Sorry about that,' she said. 'Another five minutes and the phone would have been switched over to Caredoc. You would have been heading home knowing nothing about it.'

Caredoc, the out-of-hours GP co-operative that had been set up a few years previously, was probably the single biggest development for country doctors in that it significantly reduced our on-call commitment. Nonetheless, once I knew about a call, I would not leave it for Caredoc, even if it was already six o'clock. In any case, I was one of the few people Miss Durkin would allow into her house, a house that she herself had not been out of in over thirty years.

As a younger doctor, I would have been flattered by being among the favoured few, but I had learned to be wary of those who wanted only me, knowing how easy it was to drown in the unreasonable expectations and relentless demands of highly dependent patients. I had become better at spotting the early warning signs. There was no need for such vigilance with Miss Durkin, however. She was an undemanding 83-year-old, who rarely contacted the surgery, but when she did, it was always to ask for a visit.

As a GP registrar in Derbyshire, I had loved house calls. I would take my list of people to visit and set off in the early afternoon, taking my time, enjoying the scenery, listening to the car radio, before calling to a neat little house in a neat little village, occupied by an even neater little old man or woman, who needed a repeat prescription or had to have their blood pressure checked. Even the country lanes had names in Derbyshire and all the houses were numbered in a logical sequence. Doing house calls in Tipperary was not like that. There never seemed to be enough time. I was always getting lost on country lanes, wrecking my shoes in mucky farmyards and gingerly making my way past unfriendly dogs. At least Miss Durkin did not have a dog, I thought, as I determined that I would be in and out of there as quickly as possible.

Bridget Mary Durkin, who was always known as Miss Durkin, lived alone in a secluded farmhouse a few miles outside of town. Her father had been a prosperous farmer and her mother, a teacher in the local school. She was the youngest of three daughters. All three girls had been sent to boarding school in the expectation that they would eventually become nurses or teachers. Theirs was a house of plenty. Bridget had graduated from UCD with an honours degree in politics and history. After graduation she'd gained employment as a personal secretary to an eminent barrister-at-law in Dublin. The rumour in the town was that she had been married to a fellow law student but that he had died in tragic circumstances early in their marriage and she had never re-married. I never asked her about this and she never volunteered any information on that subject. I was not convinced of the veracity of that story, anyway, as she liked to be called 'Miss' and Durkin was her family name. From what I could gather, she had continued working in Dublin until her retirement, after which she'd returned to live with her parents in the farmhouse that I was going to visit, her original home. She never spoke about her sisters and I never felt I had the right to ask.

By the time I came into her life, she was living in Proustian seclusion. Despite her eccentricities, I found her to be a warm and interesting character. She exuded an aura of fading elegance and had an intelligent and determined mind. I had won some small medical victories, like persuading her to take vitamin D, because she was not getting any sunshine and was at risk of osteoporosis, but I had never managed to get her to discuss how she had come to live in such isolation and why she would not leave her house. Although she spoke very little about her own family, she frequently enquired about mine, asking what ages my children were, what class they were in in school and whether I thought any of them would ever do medicine.

Her living conditions contrasted sharply with the normality of her conversation. Diogenes syndrome is a rare disorder, named after the Greek philosopher Diogenes, which I had only ever read about in my psychiatry textbooks, but Miss Durkin exhibited four of the commonest components of the condition: self-neglect, domestic squalor, compulsive hoarding of rubbish and social withdrawal. The farmhouse was cold and dismal, the windows mysteriously dark and hollow on approach, with only ever one weak light visible from a bare bulb in a front room. Ragged and stained full-length curtains hung like sails at half-mast on the windows of what would once have been the parlour. This was where she usually received me. Through the half-open door of the room opposite I had once seen black bags stuffed with old clothes strewn amidst papers, food wrappers, broken furniture and cardboard boxes. Old newspapers, magazines and letters were piled high along the walls and covered the surface of every counter, dresser and occasional table.

When she was expecting me, she would leave the door ajar so that I could walk straight in. 'Hello,' I would call from the sunless hall, dank and musty, even on the brightest day of summer. 'It's only me, the doctor.'

'Come on in,' would come the weak but welcoming reply from the cluttered room on the right. There I would find her, sitting contentedly by the fire in a low armchair, her small, frail frame barely visible beneath her blanket. Her face was soft and pale in the firelight, hands folded in her lap, hair tied in a bun at the back of her head. She always wore the same style of skirt, blouse and cardigan, with an extra shawl around her shoulders in the colder months. This shawl was the only sign of the changing seasons.

Making my way through the debris I would join her at the fire, settling myself as best I could on an equally low armchair reserved for her few carefully chosen visitors. There were no personal photographs, no meaningful ornaments, no treasured gifts from nieces or nephews. There was no sign that she had ever been part of a loving family. She seemed to exist in a vacuum, bearing little resemblance to the intelligent daughter of wealthy parents who had lived an independent working woman's life and who had once been in love with a young law student.

The sight of the little bowls of blue pellets placed strategically adjacent to small and large holes in the skirting disturbed me the most. I had tried repeatedly to overcome my fear of rodents, using my own forms of behaviour therapy, but had not succeeded. At one time, I remember standing in front of a glass case that housed stuffed rodents in the Natural History Museum in Dublin. In a determined attempt to rid myself of this fear, I had reached out my hand to touch the glass, but I was no match for the physiological flight response that this evoked. Despite my determination, my pulse rate increased, my breathing grew shallow, my logical reasoning shut down and the muscles of my legs performed an involuntary, co-ordinated action that had me out through the front door in seconds. Later, I thought that perhaps my own irrational fears helped me to understand and accept Miss Durkin's seemingly illogical refusal to leave her house.

When I got to her house on that particular occasion, the front door was wide open and Lena, her neighbour, was waiting anxiously in the hallway. Lena came out to me and began to speak in a hurried voice, 'We found her on the floor at about five o'clock this evening,' she began. 'She doesn't know how long she has been there, but she is very cold and I was afraid to move her, in case she had broken anything.'

I pulled my coat tighter around me, feeling the cold even more after the warmth of the car, reaching in to the back seat to get my doctor's bag, before following Lena back to the house. Lena began talking again. 'I tried so often to persuade her to get a panic button that she could press, in case something like this happened. She could have linked it to my house. But you know what she is like, Doctor. She will not do anything she doesn't want to.'

'I know,' I replied. 'She has a mind of her own alright.'

'I called my son when I found her,' Lena said. 'He is upstairs with her now. We have just covered her as best we can to try and warm her up.'

'Upstairs?' I repeated, with disbelief. 'You're not telling me that she goes up and down that stairs every day?' I had always assumed that Miss Durkin had a bedroom downstairs, but I had never asked to see it. In fact, I don't think I had ever really thought about where she slept and silently reprimanded myself for this. If it had not been for the blue pellets, I might have investigated her living conditions a bit more. But now was not the time for self-recriminations.

Lena led the way through a door at the end of the hallway that gave way to a steep, narrow, and badly lit staircase. The floorboards were partially covered with a faded carpet and creaked under our weight as we ascended. I noted with dismay the absence of bannisters or handrails. As I entered her bedroom, I felt like a detective at a crime scene. The smell of mothballs and disinfectant was almost overwhelming. A double bed stood in the middle of the room, strewn with old coats and threadbare blankets. A tall oak wardrobe stood along one wall, the mirrored doors badly reflecting the light from the single naked bulb illuminating the uninviting space. A similar oak dressing table that stood facing the bottom of the bed was covered in old newspapers, junk mail, catalogues and political flyers. Stacks of papers and magazines covered the floor. Old clothes spilled out of cardboard boxes and plastic bags. A commode stood in another corner of the room. One two-bar electric heater was the only obvious source of heat and it was plugged in and placed as close to the bed as the lead would allow. Turning off her light each night, Miss Durkin would have had to make her way through this obstacle course to the bed, in darkness. I felt my irritation return. Why was she living like this and where were her family that they could not do something about it? Why had I never investigated the upstairs before? I would almost certainly have reported it to social services or at least contacted her nephew, her only known relative, to get a room renovated downstairs. This was not the time to be irritated, however. I pulled myself back to the present.

Miss Durkin lay on the floor beside her bed, covered with blankets, propped up on a pile of discoloured pillows and cushions. A man was sitting on the floor beside her, a cup of tea in his hand, trying to persuade her to take a sip. It was Lena's son, Jim. I nodded to him briefly before focusing my attention on my patient. She looked cold, frail and frightened. Despite her vulnerability she gave me a stubborn and determined look. 'You need not have come,' she said in a polite, but firm, voice. 'I'm not going to hospital, I would just like to be put back into bed, please, and I will be fine by morning.'

I couldn't help but admire her resolve, but I could be just as obstinate and broken bones or not, she was not going to stay here one night longer. However, experience had taught me that it was best not to engage in any sort of bargaining until I had the chance to think and formulate some sort of a plan. So I ignored her remark, placed my doctor's bag on the floor and knelt down beside her. 'Would you mind if I just checked you over first before getting you back to bed, just to make sure you haven't broken anything?' I asked, as I took off my gloves and stuffed them in my pocket. She didn't reply, but neither did she resist my advances.

There on the floor of the dimly lit room, I examined her, beginning with her pulse and blood pressure. This was a ritual that was familiar to both of us. As I held her frail wrist in my hand, I felt her relax a little, but her fingers were blue with cold and her pulse was weak and thready. Gradually, I moved to her lower limbs, observing the position of her legs, looking for the tell-tale sign of a fractured hip: a shortened leg with an outwardly rotated foot. Thankfully, both legs looked the same length, with feet lying in the correct anatomical position, so I proceeded to gently palpate and move the hips, watching her face for any betrayal of pain. She remained expressionless. Finally, I covered her up again as best I could and sat back on my heels. The cold was seeping in through my boots and tights and I wanted to put my gloves back on. I had to get her out of there to somewhere warm.

'OK,' I said with a smile, 'miraculously, you don't seem to have broken anything. So let's see if we can get you back to bed.'

This news was greeted with her usual equanimity. It took three of us to get her back onto the bed, lifting her small frame carefully and making her as comfortable as we could in the circumstances. Lena found a woolly cardigan among a pile of old clothes in the bottom of the wardrobe and placed it around her shoulders before tucking the blankets in around her feet, commenting that they felt cold through the thin fabric of her tights.

I was silent, wondering how I was going to get her out of here to a warmer, safer place. Jim had slipped away after asking if I needed him for anything else. Both Lena and Miss Durkin were, by then, looking at me expectantly. What was I going to say? What was I going to do?

Taking a deep breath, I sat on the edge of the bed and covered her pale, thin hand with mine. 'You can't stay here.' I said as kindly as I could. 'Much and all as I don't want to move you out of your home, I don't see any way that you can stay. You won't be able to get in and out of bed on your own, never mind get up and down the stairs.'

There was no reaction. I would have understood tears, or pleading, or both, but she remained silent before turning away and withdrawing her hand from mine. 'I am going to call an ambulance,' I went on, feeling in my pocket for my phone. 'I will ask them to take you to the local hospital. They will take good care of you there.'

'Can I have a word, doctor,' Lena asked, making her way out to the landing and indicating that she would like me to follow. I turned and followed her out, reassuring Miss Durkin that I would be back in a minute.

'She won't go, you know,' said Lena. 'I don't know what you are going to do with her, but I know she won't leave this house. The last time she fell, we called the ambulance, but when it arrived, she refused to get into it. She clung to that bed screaming and we just couldn't persuade her to go. She will never leave here except in a box.'

'Well, I can't leave her here,' I said. 'She will die of hypothermia. I'm half-frozen myself and I'm only here half an hour or so.'

Lena left, offering to come back later if I needed her. I noticed she was shaking her head as she went down the stairs, probably wondering which of us was the more stubborn. Lena might be able to call later and while it was a kind offer, allowing Miss Durkin to remain at home was not an option. She would need a lot more support than one neighbour and she was unlikely to allow anyone else into the house. And I could not be expected to call every day to make sure she was OK: there were limits to my time and availability. Before I re-entered the bedroom, I rang the ambulance.

'I have a plan,' I said, when I went back into the bedroom. 'I am not sending you to hospital, but I want you to consider another possibility.'

Her reply was a piercing scream, followed by loud sobbing. She curled herself into a ball and turned away from me. I had never seen her like this. She was not recognisable as the dignified lady who would sit amidst the squalor and talk of her days in Dublin. 'No, no, no,' she screamed repeatedly, her voice stronger than I had ever heard it. 'I will not go, I will not go.'

Once I had recovered from the shock of the sudden outburst, I pressed on. I remembered doing a house call with a consultant psychiatrist when I started my GP training. The lady we were visiting was convinced that her neighbours were tracking her thoughts through a bug they had placed in her house. Rather than trying to convince her that this was not true, the psychiatrist had worked with her delusion, saying he believed her and would be keeping a close eye on the proceedings, persuading her to take medication for the additional stress that this was putting her under. He had also checked the house for suspicious-looking wires. 'You can never be certain,' he'd said to me as he'd looked in the cupboard under the kitchen sink.

To this day, I am not sure if he was serious, or simply wanted me to understand the importance of convincing the patient that he was taking them seriously. It was his kindness and ability to connect that I remembered. It was these skills rather than any superior medical knowledge that had allowed him to help that woman. I tried this approach with Miss Durkin now. Ignoring the screams, I agreed with her that the world outside her home was a very frightening place, but I trusted that she would manage to adjust to it. I told her that she deserved to be warm and safe and that I was going to organise for her to go someplace for a short time to receive the care she deserved. Her house had become unsafe. Her home was no longer a suitable refuge. It was time to find another.

'You have to trust me that this is the best thing for you,' I said. 'You should know me well enough by now to understand that I would not do anything that wasn't in your best interest.' Gradually, I began to feel as if I was in charge, as if her resistance was weakening. The screams stopped, but she still would not look at me. Sitting back down on the side of her bed I laid my hand on hers, which was still cold. She did not pull it away.

'You don't have to go to hospital,' I said. 'I might be able to get you a bed in the nursing home, just until you feel you can get back on your feet again.' I don't know why I said this. There were never any free beds in nursing homes and even if there were, the regulations insisted that mounds of paperwork be submitted, months in advance of securing one. In all my years of working as a GP, I had never organised an 'emergency' nursing home admission. I don't know why I thought I could do it then, but there were no other alternatives.

She turned towards me, as if considering this possibility.

'I will go with you,' I said, while I had her attention. 'And make sure that you are settled in before I leave.' I had witnessed her fear and, at some level, it resonated with me. There might not have been any rational basis for it, but it was real and terrifying for her. 'I'll just ring the nursing home and see if they have a bed,' I said, after a few minutes of silence.

'How far away is it?' was her only reply.

The nursing home I had in mind was about fifteen minutes from her house. I rang and asked for the owner, who was still on the premises despite the late hour.

'We'll find a bed,' she said, after listening to my story. 'And if Miss Durkin agrees to stay, we can sort the paperwork later.'

I heard the ambulance pull into the yard below and by the time I got down the stairs, the driver and his companion had already got out and were coming through the door, which was still wide open. A low wailing sound came from upstairs. I introduced myself to the two men, while trying to ignore the sound.

'Chair or stretcher?' the younger of the two asked, turning back towards the ambulance.

'Stretcher,' I replied.

While he was gone, I explained the situation to his partner as concisely as I could.

'I'm sorry, doctor,' the man said, when I had finished. 'I'm afraid we are not authorised to bring people to nursing homes. We were told it was the hospital.'

I had half-suspected that this might be a problem. As with most public services, there are rules and regulations and they don't always allow for the unexpected. The wailing was getting louder.

'It sounds like she might need to go to hospital in any case,' he said. 'She sounds like she is in pain.'

'That sound you hear is fear,' I said, with as much restraint as I could muster. 'She is terrified at the thought of leaving her house and adamant she will not go to hospital. Apparently, she had a bad experience there many years ago. I have managed to get her to agree to go to the nursing home, but only if I go with her and if we go without too much fuss or delay. I cannot leave her here on her own, as there is no one to come in and look after her.' I paused to check that he was still listening. 'I know there are rules and regulations, but I am asking for your help to do the only humane thing I can think of tonight. If you insist on her having to go to hospital, I will have to send her against her will and she will have to be declared of unsound mind. That will involve invoking the Mental Health Act and I really don't want to do that.'

The ambulance driver shook his head slowly, obviously weighing up his options. His partner had joined us with the stretcher and caught the end of the conversation. They looked at each other wordlessly. I looked away, not wanting to appear desperate or confrontational. It was important for GPs and ambulance crews to understand each other, to observe the professional boundaries and to respect each other's limitations. They would have to explain themselves to their line managers. They couldn't just go about depositing people at all sorts of undesignated places. I could understand that. I hoped they could understand this unorthodox situation and the need for an unorthodox solution.

'Right so, Doc,' said the older man, 'let's get this show on the road. The nursing home it is.'

I heaved a sigh of relief. To this day, I am grateful to these men for their decision to turn a Nelson's eye to the protocols and manuals and do the right thing. I am not sure how they explained it back at base.

Back in the bedroom, Miss Durkin had pulled the blankets up over her head and was sobbing loudly. I indicated to the ambulance men to stay at the doorway, while I went in and shifted the papers off a chair and dragged it to the side of the bed. I gently lifted the blanket from her head and bent down close to her. 'The ambulance crew are here,' I said slowly. 'There are two men and they are going to get you on to a stretcher and into the ambulance and then to the nursing home.'

She covered her face with her hands and continued sobbing and trembling as they moved her from the bed. Once on the stretcher, she grabbed my arm with both hands, pulling me closer to her. I gently pulled the blanket up over her head and in this manner, we proceeded to the stairs.

At the top of the stairs I prised myself away from her and said I would go down ahead and be there for her when she got to the bottom. She let out a piercing cry that startled the two ambulance men, who looked at me questioningly. 'Just keep on going down,' I advised. 'She will be OK, once we get moving.'

Miss Durkin never returned to her farmhouse again. Her first three days in the nursing home were difficult for her and the staff. She imagined everyone was her enemy and cried whenever anyone came near her. Despite this, the kindly staff managed to wash and dress her and settle her in. As the weeks went by, she became more and more relaxed and trusting, gradually getting to know the nurses and catering staff, asking them about their families and even talking to other residents. I was very happy with her achievement and could not help but silently congratulate myself for the part that I had played in it. The nursing home was a much better place for her than her miserable home.

For the first few weeks I stayed away. I was afraid that if she saw me, she would ask me if she could go home and, like a mother whose child is not keen on staying in school, I didn't want to disturb her settling-in process. When eventually, I did go to visit her, she seemed pleased to see me. I ventured to ask her if she was happy and felt safe again.

'I am,' she replied. 'I am well looked after here. It is easier on me and the nurses are very nice.'

'So, do you think you will stay, then?' I went on, feeling confident that she would now say yes.

'I probably will, doctor,' she said. 'It was cold in that house and I don't think I could get used to that again.'

'That's good,' I replied. She seemed back to herself, as she was when I used to visit her in her front room, sitting either side of the fire. 'Do you mind if I ask you one more question?' I asked then. 'It's just been on my mind for a while and I wanted to know what you think.'

'Of course, Doctor,' she replied.

'I'm just wondering what you would want me to do if you became suddenly ill and you were unable to tell me what you wanted. Would you want to go to hospital, or would you want to stay here and not have any further treatment?'

Miss Durkin might have had irrational fears, but there was nothing wrong with her day-to-day thinking. As far as I was concerned, she was capable of saying what she wanted with regard to her own healthcare and it was up to us, her carers, to respect her wishes, if at all possible. There was nothing indecisive about her reply. 'I don't care how sick I get, Doctor,' she said, 'I never want to go to hospital. I am old enough to die. I will be happy to go when my time comes.'

'OK,' I responded. 'I will write that in your file. I can always alter it later, if you change your mind.'

I was relieved to have that sorted and that everyone would know her wishes. She was, by then, almost 84 years of age and it was reasonable to accede to this last wish. She was, indeed, old enough to die. There would be no heroic measures to prolong life. When her time came, she wanted to go peacefully in this, her final home, without too much medical intervention and I was confident that we would be able to do this for her.

One Monday morning, a couple of years later, Angela stuck her head around my door, just as I was preparing for the morning surgery. 'Did you hear that Miss Durkin died at the weekend?' she asked.

'Oh, no, I didn't,' I said. 'It must have been fairly sudden. I saw her a couple of weeks ago and she was fine. Do you know what happened?'

'I don't know all the details, but the nursing home rang this morning. They said she got a pain in her chest on Friday night, but didn't want them to call the doctor. She was worse on Saturday morning, so they insisted on getting the emergency doctor out. Apparently, he took one look at her and sent her in.'

I was on my way to the kitchen as she spoke, but her words made me stop in my tracks. 'In where?' I asked.

'Clonmel, I think,' Angela replied, thinking I was asking which hospital she went to.

'But where in Clonmel?' I insisted, although I already knew the answer. 'Not the hospital? Please don't tell me she was sent to hospital.'

'Well, of course it was the hospital. Where else would they send her?'

'Damn, damn, damn!' I repeated, not caring that patients had started to file into the waiting room and could hear me.

'What's the matter?' Angela enquired, following me into the kitchen and closing the door behind her. 'What's wrong with sending her to hospital?'

'What's wrong is that it was her one wish that she would never have to go to hospital and I more or less promised her that, no matter what happened, I would not send her.'

'Oh, I see,' she said.

Miss Durkin's final journey bothered me all day. Eventually, I rang the owner of the nursing home to see what exactly had happened. She said that Miss Durkin had been in a lot of pain and that the emergency doctor had not been happy to leave her, fearing that she might get worse overnight. It had happened so suddenly. There was only one nurse on and she could not have managed Miss Durkin and all the other patients. Of course, I understood their predicament, and the decision had to be made that would be in the best interests of all.

'She didn't protest,' the owner said. 'She was too ill.'

I hoped that was the case. I hoped she hadn't felt the fear I had witnessed earlier on her last journey. I hoped she hadn't felt betrayed by those she had trusted. I wished that she had died peacefully in her bed, in the company of people who cared for her. But real-life stories have a way of saving us from complacency, with their not-so-happy endings, and I would have to live with the unsettling feeling of failure that this one had engendered in me, in the hope that any lesson learned would help me achieve better endings for others in the future.

CHAPTER FOURTEEN

UNFINISHED STORIES

After a time, I came to terms with Miss Durkin's story. At least I knew the ending, even if it was not the ending that I had wished for her. I had to remind myself that there were life stories that did have happy outcomes, but there were also many times when I did not know the outcome of a particular story that had been shared with me in the privacy of the consulting room. As a person who likes her stories to have a beginning, a middle and an end, that was something that I found particularly challenging. I would often find myself thinking about a particular patient and wondering if my words and actions had helped; if my advice had fallen on deaf ears; if it been the correct advice, or if I would change it in hindsight.

It was common for patients to find themselves in the consulting room completely overwhelmed or paralysed by a personal, family, relationship or financial crisis, with no idea what exactly they thought I could do for them. As the first point of contact for many people and the gatekeeper to many other services, it was up to me to help them make sense of what they were experiencing and to present a possible path forward, or at least point them towards a place where they could rest for a while until they figured out their next step. Sometimes, I never saw these people again, but their stories stayed with me, like a half-finished novel left behind on a train, and I had no option but to imagine the many possible endings.

Margaret's story was one of those that, for years, I had hoped had a happy ending. The first and only time I saw Margaret in the surgery, she was wearing a perfectly tailored, camel-coloured wool coat over a fitted, deep-burgundy dress and knee-high, tan leather boots with a medium heel. She looked as if she might have come straight from a fashion shoot. Her hair was cut short in a modern style, brown, with subtle highlights. Her make-up was flawless. Well, not entirely flawless, as her mascara was just the tiniest bit smudged. She looked to be in her early forties and apart from the very minor mascara indiscretion, she gave an impression of style, confidence and money.

She took her seat in the patient's chair while I closed the door after her and, even before I sat down, I felt suddenly dumpy and shabby and markedly underdressed by comparison. My vintage cardigan with its delicate pearl buttons and my straight, beige linen skirt that I had put on that morning without too much thought, seemed dated and cheap and crumpled. Over the years, I had developed my own dress code: not too casual, to help me exude some level of competence, but not too formal either, so that patients would not feel they were at a job interview. My clothes needed to be comfortable and practical because in the course of a day, I could find myself climbing over fences to get to a hunting accident, or picking my way through a muddy farmyard. In Margaret's presence, my internal narrative became harshly self-critical. Up until the minute I'd seen Margaret get up from her seat in the waiting room, I had been completely unaware of my physical appearance and had been going about my day unselfconscious and at ease. I was disturbed by how easily I had started to beat myself up.

However, I did not have time to ponder that then. I put myself, my internal narrative and my feelings to one side and gave Margaret my full attention. As I did, I noticed that not only was Margaret's mascara a little smudged, but her eyes were red, as if she had been crying or had not slept the night before. And there was something else about her that I could not put my finger on at the time, but as the consultation progressed, I suspected was fear. She seemed to be surrounded by an invisible, but palpable veil of it. Something, or someone, was threatening her and she was struggling to tell me what it was, but I had not spoken, except to call her name in the waiting room, I was not her usual GP and it was her first time attending the practice.

I continued to resist the urge to speak. I had a feeling that I would serve her best by remaining silent, that her story would gradually appear, like a painting on a blank canvas, building layer upon layer and that I should not make any judgement or assessment until I could see a clearer picture. The clock on my desk continued to measure out the passing of time, the second hand moving silently but steadily on its defined course. Normally, I used that second hand to count the patient's pulse, but that day, it reminded me only that seconds were passing, and I decided that I would speak if Margaret was still silent after a minute. Thirty seconds passed and she remained silent and did not raise her head to make eye contact. Still I did not speak, or cough, or move, or click on my computer, even though I wanted to. I had no idea what she was about to tell me, but whatever it was, I knew it was more than a sore throat, a chesty cough or a repeat smear test.

She sat upright, hands on her lap, her fingers tightly interlaced, burgundy nail varnish that matched her dress on her perfectly manicured nails. Eventually, she looked up and our eyes met. Her speech, when it did come, was matter of fact, her voice surprisingly steady, her eyes dry, but alert and fearful. 'I'm here about my daughter,' she said. 'I think she has anorexia.'

I was not expecting this. I had been bracing myself for domestic violence, for an unfaithful partner or a concern about possible cancer. I felt my heart sink a little. I knew enough to understand, that if a mother had come to the conclusion that her daughter had anorexia, there was a high probability that she was correct. And if she was, they both had a long and arduous journey towards recovery.

Nobody wants a diagnosis of anorexia, a cruel and relentless eating disorder that has the potential to destroy a person's life, robbing them of their personality, their sense of purpose and meaning, their ability to think logically, their right to pleasure and joy. Nobody wants to speak the word 'anorexia' in the same sentence as 'my daughter'. The year was 2008 and the services for a child with anorexia were limited. Even among the medical profession, there was little understanding of the causes of this disease and among the public there were many misconceptions. Some considered it a disease of celebrities, female models and actresses who chose to starve themselves in order to look good and remain successful. Others associated it with bad parenting, with over-controlling mothers, trauma or abuse. I was not a psychiatrist or a psychotherapist, no matter how many books I had read, but I did not subscribe to either of those camps. My understanding of an eating disorder was of a complex disease with dangerous consequences, which visited all manner of people, male and female, from all sorts of backgrounds and families. Evidence for the role of genetics was just emerging and it was a much more believable explanation than that of bad parenting. In my mind, an eating disorder was a disease like diabetes, asthma or depression, where genetics loads the gun and environment pulls the trigger. Treatment needed to be rational and evidence-based, but in 2008, this was not easy to access in Ireland.

But the consultation was not the place to bemoan the lack of services: I had an opportunity to make a difference for this one family and I did not want to waste that opportunity. 'Tell me a bit more,' I said. I needed to hear her story and I knew it was going to be a long and difficult one.

Margaret hesitated, as if she were sorry that she had spoken. As if speaking the words out loud had only just made it true. I wondered if this was the first time that she had said that sentence aloud, 'I think she has anorexia', and how it must feel to say that. I imagined she must want to leave, to rewind the scene, go backwards out the door and start again, take back her words, play a different DVD. I imagined she wanted to say, 'Sorry, Doctor, I don't know what came over me or what made me say that. I must have been dreaming. My daughter is fine. I'm just here for myself.'

But that was not possible. She had crossed the Rubicon and there was no going back. She had to tell her story. What she managed to say next was a weak attempt at an escape, however. 'I'm probably wasting your time, doctor. I wanted my daughter to come and see you, but she refused. She said it was me who needed the doctor. Maybe she is right. Maybe I have myself all worked up over nothing.'

I couldn't let her off the hook, even though a part of me wanted to do just that, for both our sakes. Instead, I sat forward, leaning towards her, my elbows resting on my desk, my fingers interlaced, mirroring hers, which were still resting on her lap, but not so tightly bound together as when she'd first come in. 'I'm glad you came,' I said. 'You have done the right thing. Just tell me in your own time what has been going on.'

Margaret described the almost imperceptible decline in her fourteen-year-old daughter's mental and physical health over the previous two years. Her daughter Ann, had been a happy, bright, fun-loving twelve-year-old, full of life and joy and energy, but that seemed so long ago that she hardly remembered it. It was only in her sleep, when she dreamt that Ann was her old self, eating freely, talking and laughing with friends, that she got any relief from the sense of despair and hopelessness that accompanied all her thoughts about her daughter. Ann's friends no longer came to their house. Her schoolwork had deteriorated. Her teachers had called Margaret in to see if there was anything wrong at home, as Ann had become withdrawn and was not sitting with her friends at lunch- and break-time, preferring instead to sit alone or go for a walk around the playing fields. On a couple of occasions, Ann had been in the gym during a free period when she should have been studying. At home, she was moody, argumentative and spent a lot of time looking at cookery programmes. She avoided mealtimes, saying she was sick or full or had eaten earlier. Margaret had asked her own friends who had older children what she should do, but they'd told her it was 'just a phase, they all go through it'. They'd advised her not to make a fuss, but Margaret could feel Ann slipping further and further away from her and she wanted to pull her back before she was beyond reach.

I had heard more than enough to know that Ann had an eating disorder. The question was, how was I going to help them both? Two years earlier, I had referred a young girl with an eating disorder to the Child and Adolescent Mental Health Services, CAMHS, as it is commonly known. Eventually, after about 18 months of treatment, she was discharged, deemed cured, but her mother had a different story, one of cyclical food restriction, of bingeing and vomiting. Her symptoms were no better after discharge than when she had first been referred. But I was jumping ahead of myself. As always, when I was faced with a complex problem that required time and expertise, I tried to deal with it in bite-sized chunks, to lay a path for myself and the patient that we could both follow until they were once again back on their own individual track. It was time to carve that path. Margaret had come to me looking for guidance. I was not going to solve any of her problems that day, but I wanted to make sure that when she left, she had at least a sense of hope.

I gently confirmed that, based on what Margaret had told me, Ann did, indeed have an eating disorder and reassured her again that she had done the right thing by looking for help. I acknowledged her sense of despair and hopelessness, but challenged it by letting her know that an eating disorder is a treatable condition, difficult, but treatable, and if she was to help her daughter, there was no room for hopelessness or despair.

Margaret interrupted me as I said this. 'But, Doctor, I feel so guilty. I keep asking myself what I did wrong. What terrible thing could have happened Ann to cause this.'

I tried to explain that there were many causes, but that the causes did not really matter to her at that time. What mattered was helping Ann to get better. I was reminded, as I spoke, that, a couple of years earlier I had accompanied Liam on a historical trip in North Tipperary. I had been only mildly interested in the history, but one of the buildings that we'd looked at was an old abbey, which had been almost completely covered in dark green ivy. Our tour guide had explained that the building had become unsafe, as the ivy had damaged the structure underneath and the historical society had employed someone to strip away the ivy and rebuild the structure, stone by stone. This was a painstakingly slow process that had to be done with care, patience and attention to detail. Stripping away too much of the ivy at once could lead to the collapse of a whole section of the building and make rebuilding much more difficult, or even impossible. The stripping and reparation had to be done in tandem. I had been reading the latest literature on eating disorders around that time and as the guide explained how the ivy damages the structure, it had struck me that that was exactly how eating disorder destroys a person's core.

I tried to explain this to Margaret, that an eating disorder is like ivy growing on a stone wall. At first, it may appear to enhance the structure, but underneath this seemingly harmless façade, it extends its tendrils and roots deep into the matrix of the wall, destabilising it, breaking it up, loosening the connections, until all that is left is the ivy itself, a façade without a core. There is no point asking why the ivy grew there. The only thing to do is to gently and firmly separate it, rebuild the structures underneath as you go and stop it spreading any more. There was no time to waste looking for a cause. There was no place for guilt. She needed to use all her resources to help her daughter overcome her illness, until Ann became strong enough to help herself.

As I spoke, I saw the despair lift, the fear loosen its grip, just a little. 'So, she can get better?' she said. It was more of a statement than a question and I thought I detected the beginning of a hopeful narrative. Building on this, I pressed forward with what I saw as other reasons to be positive: Ann was still young and living at home, so regular meals, consistent loving care and a safe environment, where she could be herself, coupled with therapy, would go a long way towards helping her recover. But first, Margaret needed to have Ann medically assessed to make sure she was not in physical danger from malnutrition. Ann should not be allowed to refuse this assessment. Margaret needed to be kind, but firm, when discussing this.

'I can do this for her, if you like, or you can bring her to your own GP,' I said. I had been wondering why Margaret had attended me and not her own GP for this, but had not felt the opportunity to bring this up until then.

'I'll ask her what she would prefer,' she replied. 'I came to you today because I felt too ashamed to see my own GP. He knows us pretty well and I just could not imagine telling him all this. I was worried he would think badly of us all and wonder if we were not the family he thought we were.'

I reassured her that eating disorders were common and that every GP would care for such families. No GP would judge her or blame her for the fact that her daughter had developed it, but if she really did not want to see her own GP, I would do it and she and Ann could decide what to do after that. After her medical assessment Ann would need to be referred for therapy, but with the proper treatment and help, she could make a complete recovery.

I sounded more optimistic than I felt when it came to treatment. I assumed, from Margaret's appearance and life history, that she had the means to pay for private treatment for Ann. She was lucky that Ann was young and living at home, but her age also put her at a disadvantage. Many private treatment centres were staffed by adult psychiatrists and were not licensed to treat anyone under the age of eighteen. CAMHS was the only public service for adolescents in the country, the waiting lists were long and they were not necessarily staffed with people who had experience of treating eating disorders, although most CAMHS workers had some training in this area. In-patient treatment was reserved for the dangerously physically unwell, but no child should be allowed become that unwell before accessing treatment. From what I had gleaned from Margaret, Ann was not that physically ill, which was another reason to be positive, but not a reason to delay treatment.

The consultation had run a long way over time and I thought that we were about to finish when Margaret started to speak. 'Doctor, I know you said that I should not be hung up on a cause and that I should not feel guilty, but do you think I have in some way contributed to this?' Margaret described how she often complained about her weight and that whenever she got together with female friends or family, someone would always bring the conversation around to weight and diets and food. There was always someone in the company who never felt slim enough or attractive enough and who gave out to themselves for eating whatever it was they were eating. She worried that this was what had sparked Ann's illness.

I advised her that it would be best if people did not talk about food and body shape and diets in Ann's company, but that this was not the cause of her illness. Women will continue to feel body dissatisfaction and it will affect their quality of life, but not all will develop an eating disorder. It takes a particular cocktail of ingredients for this to develop. I suggested that she should try be kind to herself and her daughter and not try to figure out too much. That her resources would be low due to the chronic stress she was experiencing as a result of Ann's illness and that she herself was not the cause, but a very necessary part of the solution.

Margaret left with a plan and the option of re-attending me on her own, or with Ann, if she needed to, but she never came back to the surgery. I thought of her from time to time and wondered what had happened after that day.

Three years later, on a wet February evening, I rushed into the Premier Hall in Thurles. I was there to see the musical *All Shook Up,* which was being produced by the Christian Brothers School, but which had borrowed girls from both the Presentation and Ursuline Convents for the girls' parts. One of those girls was my own daughter, Ailshe, who was in Transition Year in Presentation Convent. It was my third consecutive night at the musical. I was a bundle of nerves. My heart was pounding and my mouth was dry, my brow furrowed. Without looking right or left, I got my ticket and sat down cautiously in the first available seat. In any minute the musical would start. Ailshe would appear on the stage to sing the opening song. Or would she? After two nights of playing Natalie, the female lead, she had woken that morning unable to speak. Her voice was completely gone.

'You can't possibly sing tonight,' I'd said to her.

For once, she couldn't argue with me. She'd grabbed a pen and paper and had written heavily on it, <u>THERE IS NO ONE ELSE!</u> There was no understudy. There would be no show if she was not able to sing and all the tickets had already been sold. She'd spent the day sipping honey and lemon and had taken paracetamol. She was not ill, but by twelve o'clock that day, she still had not been able to speak.

'I'm going to ring the school,' I'd said to her, but she was adamant that she would be able to do it. She'd felt her voice improving. She had just one more night of the show to do and she could not let everyone down. 'Please, Mum,' she'd whispered. 'You have to let me do this.'

By the time her friend's mother had come to collect her for the show, she had just about managed to squeak. Now, as the curtains opened, and the orchestra started, I could not enjoy the music. I could see Ailshe in the shadows, waiting for her cue to move towards centre stage. I couldn't watch. I closed my eyes and held my breath. Then I heard it, the opening bars of 'Love Me Tender', sung in a voice clear and sweet, perfectly in tune, with only a very slight hint of the earlier hoarseness, so slight that only a mother would notice. It was a miracle. I had no idea how she had managed it.

'Thank God,' I said to myself, lifting my head and looking around me for the first time since I came in. I smiled at the lady next to me, who was looking quizzically at me. I thought she looked familiar, but could not place her. Perhaps I had met her at a parent–teacher meeting or perhaps just seen her around town. I relaxed a little in the chair. I was aware that Ailshe could still run into difficulty – she had quite a few numbers to sing yet – but I thought that she would probably manage it, even if it wasn't pitch perfect. Feeling more relaxed, I found myself wondering where I knew this lady from. She was neatly dressed in a black wool jacket, neat beige trousers and ankle boots. As she reached into her bag for a tissue, I caught a flash of pink nail varnish on perfectly manicured nails. Our meeting flashed before me. It was Margaret. She looked well and happy and relaxed. I made up my mind that I would not make myself known to her unless she recognised me.

As soon as the lights went on at the interval, she turned to me and, in a quiet voice, said, 'Doctor Gannon, you probably don't remember me. I came to see you once a few years ago.'

'Of course I remember you,' I replied. 'It's Margaret, isn't it?'

Just then, a group of girls approached from the bottom of the hall. They buzzed around Margaret. A tall, dark-haired girl seemed to be the leader of the group. 'Mam,' she said. 'Have you change of ten euro? I want to get some raffle tickets.' The girls were gone as quickly as they had arrived.

'Your daughter?' I said to Margaret.

'Yes,' she replied, smiling. 'She's great. You warned me it would be a long haul and a bumpy ride and so it was. Still is, at times, but we are all good now. Different, but better.'

'I'm glad,' I replied. 'So glad to hear that.'

As the curtain went up for the second and final act, I forgot that I had any reason to be anxious and became fully absorbed in the music and dance, relieved and a little bit sad that this was the closing night. By the time the cast sang the encore, 'C'mon

Everybody' , the whole audience was on its feet and I imagined that no one on stage was worried about their voice. As I sang along, I couldn't help but marvel at the resilience and determination of both young girls – Ann, who was overcoming a devastating illness, and Ailshe, who had been brave enough to step out on stage, knowing that she might not be able to perform. As Ailshe and I drove home, she thanked me for letting her go on stage that night and I thought about how parenting requires not only resilience, but hope and trust and the willingness to take centre stage, or to wait in the wings, whatever the situation demands.

CHAPTER FIFTEEN

AN UNCOMFORTABLE
SITUATION

Over the years, our practice has had a succession of GP registrars and there is a particular cohort of patients who like to see the young doctors. I think that this is possibly because these patients get tired of always hearing the same responses from Liam and me and imagine that the younger doctors might have new and innovative treatments for their ailments. Others claim that they feel they are a 'torment' and believe they are doing us a favour by 'tormenting' someone else, and giving us a break.

While it is good that patients have a choice of doctors, it is not good for anyone to be constantly switching from one to another. Sometimes, Liam would ask Annemarie, our latest secretary, to put a note on a patient's file to the effect that they were not to see the registrar until either he or I had seen them and got some idea of what was going on with them. It was not that these young doctors were more likely to miss something, it was that they were inclined to order tests of dubious validity, or even unnecessary tests, as they did not have the benefit of knowing the full background and history of each patient; despite meticulous and conscientious record-keeping, with larger files it was difficult to keep track of all the investigations that someone had already had.

Rebecca was our latest registrar. She was in her fourth year of GP training, which meant that she would be a fully qualified, independent GP in less than a year, having completed six years in medical school, a one-year internship in hospital, and another four years on the GP training scheme. One morning after surgery, she asked me if she could have a word. It was unusual for a registrar to come to me with a problem. Liam had taken over the role of GP trainer in the practice after I had become an assistant programme director, and I wondered what could be bothering her that she felt she could not discuss with him.

She explained that there was a particular male patient she had seen that morning, whom she did not want to see again. 'I can't say exactly why he made me feel so uncomfortable,' she said, looking very ill at ease. 'He didn't do anything, but he starting asking about boyfriends and babies and where I go for a night out and telling me I was a "fine-looking woman", and I just didn't like it. I felt I couldn't get rid of him quickly enough.'

Rebecca was a Dublin girl, who had found, to her surprise, that she was quite at home in 'rural Ireland'. Born with a naturally happy disposition, she saw the good in everyone and was always eager to be helpful. It was not like her to be so perturbed. I had a look at the patients she had seen that morning and immediately identified the man she was referring to. The first word that came to my mind was 'harmless', but I kept this to myself. The way this man behaved with me and the way in which he behaved with a new, young doctor could be very different and I did not want her to think that I was dismissing her concerns.

'You are sure he didn't actually do anything?' I asked.

'Oh no. I would tell you if he did, but I would prefer not to be alone in a room with him again. He felt a bit creepy.' She said this in a low voice, as if she was afraid of being overheard, or judged as not fit for her job.

'Of course,' I said. 'It's not a problem. Annemarie can make sure he is booked for either Liam or myself for now. She can just put a "not for reg" note on his file, but you should mention this to Liam. It might be something you could discuss in a tutorial.' In addition to 'on-the-spot' teaching, Liam met with the registrar twice weekly for formal tutorials. During these sessions, they explored the art, as well as the science, of general practice. Most registrars found that the science was the easiest part. It was things like dealing with uncertainty, managing difficult patients, caring for those who provoke uncomfortable feelings such as irritation, anger, frustration, fear or disgust, that was difficult. How can you give health advice to a man who you suspect beats his wife? How can you be kind to the mother you fear neglects her children? How do you explore a teenager's ideas, concerns and expectations, when you have a hunch that their main aim in life is to make their parents' lives as difficult as possible? All of these people present to the surgery and are deserving of the best care we can give.

'I am human and let nothing human be alien to me' is a dictum by the Roman playwright Terence that I try to live by, especially when feeling low on compassion. This is easier said than done. True compassion for people who behave in socially unacceptable ways requires constant effort.

In a country practice, it is unusual for a doctor to say to a patient, 'I don't want to deal with you any more. I don't like how you make me feel. I would prefer if you attended another doctor.' In the case of patients who made me uncomfortable I had, over the years, managed to put judgement aside and adjust my response, so that I could do what needed to be done. I had very rarely asked a patient to attend another doctor. Rebecca was fortunate that she could excuse herself from seeing this man, but anyone working alone in a country practice will understand the complexities of dealing with someone like him. Her experience was not unique to her, or to female doctors. It was something lots of GPs had experienced at some point.

More than twenty years earlier, shortly after my return from the UK as a newly qualified GP, I had arrived at a small rural health centre where I had agreed to be the locum for the day. There were no cars parked outside the small building with the sign that said HEALTH BOARD CENTRE, but the door was open, so I parked my car, collected my doctor's bag from the boot and made my way in.

A low murmur of conversation greeted me from a room to my right. As I pushed open the door the conversation stopped and all eyes fixed on me. I estimated there were between ten and fifteen people in the room. No one spoke. 'Hello,' I said, trying to sound casual and confident, 'I'm Doctor Gannon. Am I in the right place?'

A man, who looked to be in his late fifties, looked up as I entered. He was sitting in a chair that looked much too small for his large frame. Leaning forward, he rested his arms on his widespread knees with his hands joined in the space between them. My first impression was that he was taking up a disproportionate amount of space in that small room.

He answered my question with one of his own. 'Is he not here himself today, then?' As he spoke, he let his gaze travel slowly down my body, taking me in, so that I became conscious of how I must appear to this gathering: a mere girl, round-faced, with shoulder-length blonde hair, who had, shortly before, been mistaken for the doctor's daughter. I could see the disbelief on the waiting faces, and in this man's scrutinising gaze. I tightened my grip on my still-new doctor's bag, as if I were a child and this was my mother's hand.

While I stood there, thinking these thoughts, the man stayed sitting forward, his eyes continuing to move up and down my body, as if he were surveying a racehorse before considering a purchase. Any minute, I expected him to ask me to turn around so he could get a more complete view. 'No,' I said, in a defensive voice, turning away from his gaze, 'Doctor Maloney is away today and I am doing duty for him.'

A woman appeared at the door of an adjoining room. 'In here, Doctor,' she said. 'This is the doctor's room. The public health nurse is usually in that other room, but she is out on leave. I thought you might be a new nurse when you came in.'

I thanked her and made my way into the room, relieved to be away from the questioning faces and from the man's domineering presence. I placed my bag on a small desk in the middle of the room. The bag, a present from my old training practice, had become my security: whenever I felt out of my depth or lacked confidence, that bag reminded me that I had the skills to deal with all eventualities. I imagined that the bag contained all the wisdom, guidance and reassurance ever given to me by my GP trainers, and it would be many years before I replaced it with a bigger, newer model. These GPs had held my hand as I had ventured onto the skating rink of general practice. They had picked me up when I slipped and fell and, eventually, they had let me go, with the reassurance that I could go it alone. I wondered what they would have to say about my situation that day, but I had no time for reflection or self-doubt. I had a job to do and I had to get on with it. I put the man, his roving eyes and critical gaze out of my mind.

'Are you Maggie?' I asked the lady then. In my nervousness, I had completely forgotten that Dr Maloney had told me that Maggie would be there to open up the health centre and show me around.

'I am,' she replied. 'I live next door. Just come and let me know when you are finished and I will lock up. You know you have to go to his own house for the afternoon surgery?'

'Yes, thanks,' I replied, feeling distracted. I would have to concentrate on getting through the morning first.

Maggie left me all alone in the little consulting room. I was the doctor, the nurse and the secretary. I was miles from another doctor and even further from a hospital. The waiting room was full of people I did not know and, somewhere in my consciousness, there was still that man and his gaze. With any luck, I would see him early and send him on his way.

Opening my bag, I took out my stethoscope, diagnostic set, urine dipsticks and portable blood pressure monitor and set them on the desk, before surveying the room. A narrow wooden examination couch stood alongside one wall, the top of it raised in a semi-reclining position, with a tartan blanket folded on the end. There was no curtain rail or curtain, but I noticed, with surprise, that there was a telephone on the desk. I picked it up and got a dial tone. That could come in useful, I thought. There was a chair on either side of the desk, one for the doctor and one for the patient. A small stool was positioned beneath a window that looked out on the open countryside. I noticed the hawthorn hedges were already decorated with delicate white flowers, the banks beneath them speckled with early primroses. I returned to my immediate surroundings. The only other things in the room were a small sink attached to the wall with a hand towel on a hook beside it and a filing cabinet for the patient files.

I followed Dr Maloney's instructions and retrieved the key from where he had hidden it and opened the cabinet. Without a secretary to organise appointments, patients just turned up and were seen in order of arrival. The actual order was decided by the patients. After one last glance around the room, I was ready to call my first patient.

I made slow progress, as I was not familiar with the people, with their problems or their medications, but nobody seemed to mind. Most patients did not know the names of their tablets. Some reached into their pockets and produced a handful of multi-coloured pills that they set out in front of me, thinking they were being helpful, but they might as well have been showing me the contents of a packet of M&Ms, for all the good that did. I made lots of calls to the pharmacy to check on tablets.

Each time I went to the waiting room, I expected the man who had addressed me when I came in to get up and follow me to my room, but he remained sitting, seemingly in no rush, letting the older men with their walking sticks, the teenagers in their school uniforms and the frazzled mothers with their babies and toddlers in ahead of him. As the morning progressed, I became more aware of his presence, despite doing my best to avoid his gaze whenever I went out into the waiting room to call the next patient. The uneasy feeling that I had had when he first addressed me was, by then, a heavy weight on my chest. I was distracted. I couldn't concentrate on the other patients. I was not my usual, friendly, trusting self.

Finally, hearing him tell yet another mother and toddler that they could go on ahead, I decided to confront him. I drew myself up to my full height, took a few deep breaths, and went back to the waiting room. I addressed the man directly, ignoring the other patients and said loudly, 'You have been here a long time, I'm sure it must be your turn now.'

He stayed sitting, relaxed but unsmiling, in his chair. 'I'm not in any rush,' he replied. 'I have no particular place to be. I'll let Josephine here go ahead,' he said, indicating to the middle-aged woman who had her head stuck in a copy of a well-thumbed and outdated *Far East* magazine that she should follow me. He would come in in his own time. It was obvious who was in charge, who was calling the shots. I had no option but to go along with it.

By then, I was convinced that he was deliberately trying to intimidate me, even though I had had little experience of that type of behaviour. Throughout my GP-training year, I had answered the phone to patients in the middle of the night and had gone to their homes, not knowing who or what I would find there. I had set off without the benefit of Google Maps or satnav, not knowing if I would even find my way. As a student, I had foolishly hitch-hiked alone from Letterkenny to Renvyle and had never felt uneasy with the men who had given me lifts. I had narrowly escaped an assault by a patient in a busy Birmingham emergency department and had returned to work as soon as the security staff had removed the offender. I was not easily frightened or intimidated.

Perhaps it's me, I thought then. Perhaps I am getting less trusting of the world as I am getting older. I wasn't sure why, but I knew that I did not like this man's attitude. I did not like how he insisted on letting everyone ahead of him and I did not like the fact that soon, it would be just us two in the building.

Finally, we were alone and it was his turn. He came forward with hand outstretched, leaving me with no option but to take it in mine. To cover my nervousness, I apologised for keeping him, even though he had kept himself and I had nothing to apologise for.

'Oh, not at all,' he replied. 'I am in no rush. I don't mind being the last.'

'What can I do for you?' I asked, trying not to sound anxious or rushed.

'Oh, I just want you to check my blood pressure,' he said to me, making no attempt to remove his jacket, or roll up his sleeve. He stood between me and the door, even though I had indicated that he could take a seat.

Surely he has not waited three hours just to have his blood pressure checked, I thought, but that was what he had asked me to do and I was not about to look for any hidden agenda. During my training, my GP trainer had taught me not to take simple requests at face value, as they were often just a front for a more serious and complex problem. However, I had decided that this man was well capable of putting his cards on the table and if he said all he wanted was a blood-pressure check, then that was all that I was going to do. 'OK, sure, I'll do that,' I said and picked up my stethoscope.

He still made no attempt to prepare himself for a blood-pressure examination.

'You might take off your jacket for me and roll up your sleeve,' I said, busying myself looking for his file in the cabinet, reluctant to sit down, as he was still standing.

He began to undo his jacket, pausing between buttons to ask me where I was from, if I was married, if I had any children, where I lived and how I had ended up being the locum that day. I answered as concisely as possible, not wanting to appear rude, but also not wanting to encourage further personal questions. He commented that I looked young enough to be just out of school. I ignored this remark. He worked slowly and methodically, unhurried, with no indication that he was causing unnecessary delay, or that I had already been there for three hours, working without a break and that I had to leave and go to another surgery in the afternoon.

Under the jacket he wore a jumper, shirt and tie. Eventually, he removed the jacket, walked slowly to the door and hung it on a hook that I had not noticed until then. I began to think that I would never get him out. Next, he started on the jumper, removing one arm at a time, slowly pulling it over his head, before turning it the right way round and placing it carefully on the back of the chair.

I stayed standing by the filing cabinet, flicking through the files, glancing up every now and then to see how he was progressing. I was determined not show feelings of agitation, because I felt that that was what he wanted, but all the while, my heart was beating a little bit faster than usual, keeping me alert, teetering on the edge of fight or flight.

I noticed him begin to pull at his tie. 'There's no need to take that off, I said, putting his file on the desk and looking like I was ready to do the examination. 'You can just roll up your sleeve.'

'I'm not sure if it will go up,' he said. 'It's a bit tight. It might be better if I take it off.'

'No, really,' I said. 'There's no need. It doesn't matter. Have a seat, please and I will manage it.'

Finally, he did as I asked and sat down. I imagined that, by then, my blood pressure was much higher than his. Was he playing with me? I wondered. Was he deliberately displaying his power over me? Was I in danger or was I overreacting? I remember looking at the window and wishing I had had the foresight to open it, before he came in, so that if I'd needed to raise my voice for any reason someone might have heard me. Perhaps, I thought, I might even manage to climb on the stool and escape out the window to the field with the hawthorn hedges.

'Well, you certainly have lots of layers,' I said, to ease the tension and give the impression of composure or control.

'Ne'er cast a clout till May be out,' he replied, as if this was a medical fact that I should have known. Even though he was sitting down now, and separated from me by the desk, he was still positioned between me and the door. During my psychiatry training, I had been taught to always position myself between the patient and the door, as you never knew when a patient suffering from psychosis might misinterpret signals and become suddenly violent, but I had never before thought that this might be necessary in general practice.

I asked him to place his arm on the desk and positioned the sphyg, or portable blood-pressure monitor, over his shirtsleeve, the drum of the stethoscope over his brachial artery. I inserted the ear pieces into my ears and took his blood pressure. 'That's perfect,' I announced, even though, to this day, I cannot remember if it was or not. I was too nervous to pay any attention to his blood pressure. I only remember thinking that none of this consultation was about blood pressure and this man was unlikely to look for, or follow, any medical advice from me.

'You can put back on your jacket and jumper and just come back to Dr Maloney when you need your tablets,' I said, trying not to show how eager I was to get him out.

'That's good,' he replied. 'I have no need to worry so.' With that, he began the slow methodical process of putting his clothes back on.

As I let him out, I heaved a sigh of relief. Alone at last in the health centre, my pulse slowed, my breathing deepened and I regained my equilibrium. 'You were definitely overreacting,' I said to myself, before gathering my things and going to Maggie to tell her I was finished.

Later that night I rang Dr Maloney to let him know how I got on. 'Mr D–,' I said. 'What's the story with him?' I explained that he had waited all morning to see me, had taken for ever to get undressed, and had not really wanted anything from me after all that. I did not tell Dr Maloney how ill at ease I had been in the man's presence, or that I felt intimidated by him. It did not seem important by then. I did not want him to think that I was easily frightened, or that he was wrong to have thought me capable of doing his locum.

'Oh, he's a relatively new patient,' he said. I haven't really got a handle on him yet. Was he OK with you?'

'Not a bother,' I replied. After all, he had not done anything that I could name as wrong or inappropriate, but I would certainly not want to be in his company again.

Even today, I find it difficult to say exactly what it was that I found intimidating about this man. His look, his voice, his presence, his pushing the boundaries of the doctor–patient, male–female relationship – but I was willing to believe that what Rebecca was describing was not imagined and I was glad that at least she felt safe enough to voice it.

A couple of months later, as I was coming back from lunch, I spotted Rebecca climbing over the fence that ran along the side of the surgery. From the little I saw, it was obvious that she was not a regular fence-climber. 'Communing with nature in your lunch hour?' I said, once she was back on solid ground.

She let out a startled cry and accidentally dropped her phone. 'You gave me a fright,' she said, 'sneaking up on me like that.'

'You know me, I can turn up anywhere,' I replied. 'Always on the prowl. But what were you at in the field?'

'Well,' she answered a little sheepishly, 'I was actually taking a picture of the sheep. I thought I might get a selfie, but they all ran into the corner and I had to make do with a group photo.'

She held out the phone to show me the photograph.

'Photographing sheep,' I exclaimed in disbelief. 'Anyone would think you were an American. Oh, but I forgot, you're from Dublin. Sheep are even rarer there.'

'No need for the sarcasm,' she said. 'It's not for me.' She explained that her friends could not believe that she could hear sheep outside her window as she worked and she just wanted to show them that she wasn't making it up.

'Look at that cute woolly one there,' she said, pointing at one that appeared to be looking straight at the camera.

'All sheep are woolly, unless they have been shorn,' I replied. I wondered if her friends actually realised that the leg of lamb that they had for their Sunday lunch had once frolicked around a field like this one, but I refrained from speaking my mind. Instead, I couldn't help but warn her not to oversell the country living, or we could have people arriving down from Dublin in their droves, looking to take photographs of the cute woolly sheep.

'Oh, no need to be like that. You really do have a bit of a bee in your bonnet about Dublin people,' she said. 'But on another note, you'll never guess who I saw this morning. My friend who I said I didn't want to see any more.'

I was surprised. I had forgotten all about that incident. Rebecca explained that she had answered the phone in reception earlier that morning only to find that it was her 'friend' looking for an appointment. Both Liam and I were fully booked, so she agreed to see him.

'And how did you get on?'

'Well, initially, I felt a bit uncomfortable, but when he started to veer into the personal questions, asking if I had met any nice Tipperary man to keep me warm at night, I shut him up fairly quickly. I told him I had to stick to medical matters. And that was the end of that.'

'Well done,' I said, delighted that she had embraced this challenge and overcome it, while still in the safe environment of a training practice.

I asked her what she thought was different about her second encounter with the man, that made her directly address his inappropriate remarks, and she answered that she had discussed the incident and her feelings about it with Liam. This had helped her realise that the man's comments were indeed inappropriate and that she had the power to confront him. Her comments made me think about all the women who stall at the first hurdle when it comes to addressing inappropriate workplace remarks or behaviours; who tell themselves that they are making a mountain out of a mole hill and stay silent in order not to be seen to make a fuss, as I had done all those years ago with Mr D–.

Liam was already at his desk when we went back into the surgery, checking the pile of post that had arrived that morning.

'I just found Little Bo Peep, photographing her sheep,' I said, pointing to Rebecca.

Liam looked out from over his glasses, his face grave with concern. 'You know, Rebecca,' he said, as if this was an important learning opportunity. 'There's a word for people who take pictures of sheep.'

'Oh, right,' she replied. 'And what might that be?'

'Baa … rmy,' he replied, before laughing heartily at his own joke.

Rebecca groaned. 'Not one of your better ones,' she said, with the pained expression that she seemed to reserve for Liam's jokes. It was definitely time to get back to work.

CHAPTER SIXTEEN

THIS MORTAL COIL

I had known for a long time that I would have to sort the files in the attic room in the surgery and one Saturday morning, I finally managed to motivate myself to begin. What we called the attic was a small storage room upstairs in the surgery. This room contained rows and rows of paper patient files that we no longer used, as for many years all records had been input on the computer. It had always been a requirement that medical files were not destroyed for a minimum of seven years after the death of a patient, so we had kept all patient files and had not got around to destroying any. Now, new data protection regulations were coming down the track that stated that the files of patients who had been deceased for seven years or more *had* to be destroyed. Our practice had been in operation for almost twenty years. We had a large elderly population, with a death rate of approximately twenty patients per year, which meant that there was a significant number of files to be sorted and destroyed.

As I entered the dimly lit room, I almost tripped over two large cardboard boxes that had been abandoned just inside the door. They had both been marked with RIP in bold, black letters. These were at least some of the files I was looking for, but looking at the boxes made me want to flee from the room. By then, I was used to dealing with death and dying, but those two large boxes, containing evidence of past lives, of people who had once been walking, talking and breathing, but were now gone, was almost too much to comprehend on a regular Saturday morning. Added to that was the sudden thought that life really was too short to spend my Saturday morning sorting the files of those who were beyond medical intervention, just because someone, somewhere had drawn up new regulations. The annoying quote by Annie Dillard, 'how we spend our days is, of course, how we spend our lives', came to mind and I felt damned if I did and damned if I didn't, but I had got myself as far as the attic and was drawn to at least investigate the boxes, so I carefully lifted the lid of one and peered inside, as if half-afraid that something would escape from it. I sifted through some of the files, putting to one side those of patients who had died more than seven years earlier and noting the familiar names: O'Dwyer, Murphy, Ryan and Maher. A piece of paper floated to the floor. I picked it up and glanced at the content and without warning, experienced clearly the feelings that letter had engendered in me the first time I had read it, many years earlier.

It had been an ordinary day. I was reading through the post after morning surgery. The letter I held in my hand was from an oncologist. It had read,

> 'This unfortunate man appears to have liver metastases. I have discussed the implications with himself and his wife today and they will come and see me later regarding palliative chemotherapy.'

The letter had been addressed to Liam. I'd searched for the patient's name and eventually found it, printed in small font on the top right-hand corner of the page, almost completely overshadowed by the hospital letterhead. 'Mr Dan McGuire,' it had read. I'd dropped the letter as if it were contagious. I had known the man well and that he was ill, but I had not known that he had liver metastases and that his only option for treatment was palliative chemotherapy. I'd wanted to put the letter into the shredder and pretend that it had never arrived. I could not think of that man, so full of life, as being terminally ill.

There are guidelines for doctors who have to break bad news to patients. They suggest that the doctor gives a warning shot, checks what the patient knows already, makes sure that they have somebody with them and that they are not rushed or distracted, or likely to be disturbed. I had always tried to do this when discussing bad news with patients, but as a doctor, I frequently received bad news without the benefit of these conditions. It could arrive out of the blue, as that letter had, without warning. It could be a phone call from a consultant in the middle of surgery, letting me know that someone who I had come to know and care for, and who I would have expected to be around for perhaps another twenty years, had only a few months to live. Dan McGuire was Liam's patient, so on that day I had brought the letter into Liam in his room across the corridor. Before breaking the news to him, I'd asked him if he had heard anything about Dan and warned him that the letter in my hand was not good.

'I wasn't expecting that,' Liam had said, growing quiet and thoughtful. 'I thought he might be one of the ones who was caught early. I didn't think it had spread.'

Accepting that somebody has a terminal diagnosis is never easy. When people come in to our surgery, they come as people, not patients. They step temporarily out of their own lives, leave their uncleared kitchen tables or half-weeded flower beds, to seek advice or reassurance, or to get their prescriptions renewed. They wear their own clothes, not hospital gowns or pyjamas. They share stories of their children, or grandchildren, or their next planned trip abroad. Of course, I know that many illnesses are incurable, that people of all ages die before they are ready, but in those early days of general practice, I had not yet learned to accept that these illnesses happen to people who were as engaged with living as I am. Without that acceptance, I found it difficult to care for them.

I wanted to make people better, not help them die. That was the palliative care specialists' job, when the physicians and surgeons and GPs had done all they could do. Palliative care consultants had special training. They had chosen that work freely. They were confident they could do it and do it well. I was not. But life was not like that. It was not possible to separate the living from the dying. People still lived, even while they were dying, and most wanted to do this in their own community, in the company of their families and friends. As a GP it was my job to help them do this, whether I liked it or not. No one knew these people like Liam and I did. We could get advice from specialists, but we could not hand over their care. We could not turn our backs on them in their hour of greatest need. If caring for the dying was a great sea of uncertainty for me as a doctor, I could only imagine how much more frightening a terminal diagnosis would be for patients and their families. Nevertheless, I resisted this aspect of my job, claiming lack of clinical expertise, while in reality, it was not knowledge that I lacked as much as the skills to take on the emotional labour of such work.

I put the letter back in the file and remembered the first time I had met Dan McGuire, the man referred to in the letter. Bridget had put a call through to me, saying it was urgent. I should not have been answering the phone that day, because I had taken the afternoon off to catch up on administrative work, but Liam was busy with patients. It was a Thursday afternoon and we were covering for a neighbouring GP, who took a half-day off on a Thursday.

A GP in the surgery without booked appointments is like Velcro for all manner of miscellaneous requests, so most of these 'administrative' sessions would be interrupted by phone calls or house calls, or both. The most I ever achieved on an administrative afternoon was keeping my pile of letters, reports and lab results from getting bigger. It never disappeared.

The lady on the phone said that there had been a car accident: a single car, involving one man, and asked if I could come immediately.

'Is he conscious?' I asked.

The lady answered that he was and I told her I would be out straight away, but to call the guards and the ambulance and to try not to move the patient from the car until I arrived. I briefly explained my rationale for that request by saying that even minor car accidents can result in vertebral fractures that need to be stabilised before moving.

On arrival in the village, seven miles from Killenaule, there was no sign of a traffic accident. Annoyed, I wondered if someone had decided to play a prank. I was just about to get back into my car when I noticed a man watching me from the doorway of a house on the main street. The man gestured to me furtively and I went towards him, doctor's bag in one hand, a blue trauma bag, with neck collars, intravenous lines and an oxygen cylinder, in the other.

'Are you the doctor?' the man whispered.

'Yes,' I answered, wondering who else I could possibly be, lumbering around, laden down with medical equipment.

'Follow me,' said the man, as he led me in to a house a couple of doors up from where he had been standing.

The patient, a Mr Dan McGuire, was sitting on a chair in the back kitchen of the house, smiling broadly, with a concerned group of men and women gathered around him. 'Hello, Doctor,' he said, sounding not in the least like a man who had been in an accident. 'I just had a little tip with the car. I'm fine altogether. I told them not to call you. I'm grand.'

A little tipple, more like, I thought, my annoyance abating despite myself. There was such an air of bonhomie radiating from Dan that it was difficult to be irritated.

He attempted to get up off the chair, but was quickly and gently restrained by one of the group of onlookers. 'Sit back there, Dan,' the other man said. 'Sure, the doctor was passing this way anyway. You might as well let her have a look at you, now that she's here.' The man winked at me conspiratorially from behind Dan's back.

I surveyed the scene, wondering what was going on. There was no evidence of an accident, no car and only one victim, who appeared hale and hearty, if maybe a little bit too hearty for four o'clock on a Thursday afternoon. And there was no sign of the ambulance or the guards. Part of me was relieved. At least I wasn't trying to get some poor unfortunate into a neck collar, out of a car and onto a body board.

At that point, a lady stepped forward, with an authoritative air. 'Let the doctor have a bit of space,' she said, motioning to the gathering of six or seven men to move into the front room. They did as they were told.

'I'll tell you what happened, doctor,' she said. She explained that her husband, the man I had met in the street, had been sitting at the table having a cup of tea, when he'd heard a loud noise outside the house. She herself was out the back at the washing line, so she hadn't heard it. Her husband had gone out to investigate and had seen Dan's car half in the ditch, having hit a telegraph pole at the side of the road.

'Ah, it just slipped a bit off the side of the road, doctor,' Dan interjected now. 'It didn't really crash into anything.'

The woman raised her eyebrows and told Dan to shush. He would get plenty of time to talk to the doctor when she had finished. She explained that her husband had helped Dan out of the car and had brought him in and that was when they thought they should get the doctor. They wondered if maybe he had had a little turn, like a mini-stroke, or low blood pressure or maybe even have hit his head in the crash, although there wasn't any bump or bruise.

'So where is the car?' I asked, thinking that maybe if I saw it, I could gauge the impact of the crash and see if I should be worried or not. The woman explained that one of the men had moved it around the back of another house in case anyone would see it and news of the incident would reach Dan's family before he did. I was more inclined to think that it was in case any garda happened upon it and decided to investigate it, but I kept that opinion to myself. I was the doctor, not the garda. The woman told me that she had decided that there was probably no need for the guards or the ambulance, but they'd thought it would be better if a doctor saw him before he went home. She hoped they had done the right thing.

There was nothing for it but to examine the increasingly apologetic Dan, at the end of which, I pronounced him fit to be returned to his wife, with a strict proviso that he was not to be allowed to drive his car for the next few days, until he had been re-examined by a doctor to make sure there were no delayed effects of the accident. I would be sending a note about the incident to his own GP, so that he could follow it up.

Dan cheerfully informed me that he did not have a GP. He was never sick.

'In that case,' I said, grasping the opportunity to have a cautionary word about driving under the influence, 'you can come to me or my husband, Doctor Meagher, in Killenaule. We'll be expecting you.'

Surprisingly, Dan did attend Liam the following week. As I entered the waiting room, he saw me, smiled broadly and gave me a thumbs-up, before pointing to Liam's consulting room. For the next couple of years, he attended Liam regularly. He never left the consulting room without telling a joke or a story that generated loud guffaws of laughter and that left Liam chuckling to himself long after Dan had gone.

But alongside the pleasures of getting to know patients personally, the satisfaction of feeling part of their lives and the enjoyment that I got from daily interactions with people like Dan, came the sorrow of loss when those people became seriously ill and died. As I put Dan's file in the pile to be destroyed, I could still remember the feeling of sorrow both Liam and I had experienced at his passing so many years before.

CHAPTER SEVENTEEN

COMING TO TERMS

As I continued to sort through the files of those who were gone, I remembered how unsettled I had become by some of those deaths and how I had resisted getting involved in their end-of-life care. I had searched for and found multiple reasons why Liam should provide this service and not me. Liam had not argued. He seemed to find caring for the dying easier than I did and could do so without becoming overwhelmed.

I lived with my unease for a number of years, until one day I read a quote by Ralph Waldo Emerson, which said, 'People wish to be settled; only as far as they are unsettled is there any hope for them.' This resonated with me and I thought that perhaps my feelings of unease were trying to tell me that I had resisted this aspect of care for long enough. That perhaps it was time to embrace it. As a consequence, shortly after Dan's death, I signed up for a certificate course in palliative care with the Irish College of General Practitioners. Over the course of nine months, I learned to treat the pain, the nausea and the weight loss of terminal illness. I learned what medications to use for bone pain, nerve pain, headaches and bowel spasm. I learned how to titrate, or gradually increase, the dosage of opioids so as to avoid side effects and how to diagnose and treat opioid toxicity.

I learned how to recognise when death was imminent and how to communicate this to relatives, so that they could prepare for what was to come. Gradually, I learned how to face my own fear of the finality of death and to recognise and acknowledge the grief that I sometimes felt as a doctor.

I had thought that there must be a right way for a doctor to feel, and I had not expected that to be grief. I also learned that some of my resistance had more to do with my fears and uncertainties around death than with my role as a doctor. I began to realise that it was only through facing those fears that I could be truly present for others. I learned that I was not expected to have answers to the big questions such as is there a God, a heaven or a purpose to life. In many of the houses I visited, the priest was a much more frequent presence than the doctor and even he was not expected to have answers to those questions. Some people believed in eternal life and faced their final hours with unwavering faith. Others did not and left this world satisfied that they had done the best they could. Yet others did not discuss the subject of death at all, even as I, and others, bade them a final farewell. But the greatest lesson I learned was this: it is when we decide to embrace that which we have resisted most that we experience the greatest growth and rewards.

I paused in my morning's work and realised that I had been sorting through the attic files for over two hours, completely lost in memories of earlier days. I was surprised at how easily the thoughts and feelings associated with each person resurfaced as I handled his or her file.

I made my way to the kitchenette to make a cup of coffee, but I was reluctant to leave my work, so I took the next file with me on my break. It belonged to Pat, who had died many years previously, prematurely, but in the comfort of his own home, surrounded by his family. After all the years, I could still feel the warmth of his personality from the first time I met him. This had not occurred in the surgery, however, but when he had called to our house one evening to see if he could teach me to play the accordion. A patient of Liam's, Pat was a well-known accordion player and a skilled teacher of the instrument. As far as Liam was concerned, I could already play the accordion, having learned in school: I just needed a reason and encouragement to do so. Liam never doubted my ability to do anything I set my mind to, despite the increasing assertions of my children that he was deluded. I couldn't convince him that two polkas and a jig, the only tunes I still remembered from my days in Tourmakeady, played haltingly a couple of times a year, did not make me a musician.

I owned a little black-button accordion that I had brought with me everywhere I went since my father gave it to me in my early twenties. It was a little Hohner with one row of buttons and with faded gold markings on it. It always smelled faintly of cedar and had a distinctive retro sound when played. When I was a child, this accordion was kept in the high press in the kitchen, a mysterious object that nobody except my father ever played.

'It belonged to your mother,' my father said when he gave it to me. 'Although she never played it. She wasn't very musical.'

'Why did she buy it?' I asked.

'I can't really remember,' he replied. 'I think she had it when I met her.'

My father did not talk much about my mother and we learned to treasure the memories he shared and tread lightly among them. I was content with that. He had learned to play accordion from his Uncle John, one of two bachelor uncles who lived in Cloonluane, a townland on the edge of the Renvyle peninsula, the original Gannon homestead. It was not unusual for my father to sit in the chaos of our kitchen, with the accordion on his knee, oblivious to us all, playing his own selection of tunes. I recognised many of these, but I often suspected that he made up others as he went along. Eventually, he progressed to a double-row box and the little Hohner lay abandoned and out of tune in the press until one day he entrusted it to a passing repair man, who'd breathed new life into it. Shortly after that, he gave it to me. As it was the only thing that I possessed that had belonged to my mother, I treasured it for itself, but always felt a little guilty that it was not being put to its intended use.

I opened the door for Pat on the evening of my first lesson, feeling a little nervous and self-conscious. It had been years since anyone had heard me play, apart from Liam and the kids, and I was musical enough to know that my playing was far from perfect. 'I don't know what Liam has told you,' I said to Pat. 'But I'm not very good. I haven't played in years. Not that I was any good then either and I don't even read accordion music.'

'No matter,' he replied. 'Play away, whatever you can remember.'

We were sitting in the sitting room on a bright, sunny evening. Pat settled himself into the armchair that faced out of the window and commented that the view we had of Slievenamon would inspire anyone to play music. He looked perfectly at ease and I was loath to disturb his peace with my awkward playing. But I was just making excuses. I took a deep breath and played my three Kerry polkas badly.

'Lovely,' he said when I had finished. 'You'll have no bother.' Then Pat took my accordion from me and began to play. The little accordion looked tiny on his ample lap, but there was nothing small about the sound he made with it. His fingers moved effortlessly up and down the buttons. The bellows lengthened, arched and shortened, emitting a sound that took me back to my student days, to the Crane Bar in Galway on a Sunday night, where the sound of the music mingled easily with the buzz of conversation, the clinking of glasses and the smell of whiskey and Guinness in the smoke-filled bar. The tunes were the same three polkas that I had played, with the same notes and timing, but mine had not learned to fly, while his soared and swooped and spun, way beyond my reach.

'That was beautiful,' I said, when he had finished. 'I've never heard it played like that before.'

'You'll be playing like that before long,' he said. 'With a little bit of practice every day, you'll be surprised how those tunes will take on a life of their own and you won't even know that it's you making the sound.'

Many jigs and reels and polkas later, Pat became ill and died while still in his early sixties, but his music lives on in all the pupils he taught and the recordings he made. I still have the cassette tapes he made for me. In a kind, patient and skilful way he played each tune both slowly and quickly and wrote the notes in a way that I could understand. As I placed his file on the pile for shredding, I knew he would admonish me for not continuing to play, but although I had said I would, I never found another teacher. Without Pat to encourage me and keep me motivated, I soon stopped practicing and my little accordion went back into its case where it has spent most of its time since.

After my coffee, I returned to continue my task. Lying on top of the second box was a file that had only been left there the week before. It belonged to Josephine, a woman in her late seventies, the most recent death in the practice. For the past few months, Josephine had been too unwell to come in to see me, so I had made the journey to her house at least twice a week. When she was first diagnosed with breast cancer, she had been brave and accepting: like someone standing in a line where everyone is given a heavy bundle to carry, she took hers and continued on her way, uncomplaining. 'Sure, everyone has something,' she'd said, sensing my regret and concern.

Josephine accepted all the treatments that were offered. Her follow-up scans were clear, but her worsening health indicated that something was amiss and it soon became evident that the cancer had returned. It was incurable. The specialist offered further palliative treatment and she said it would be good to have it, as she could avoid later pain and other complications. Josephine followed this expert advice, travelling the 80 kilometres to Waterford Hospital twice weekly, until she became too ill to travel. Her specialist did not say that there was no point having further treatment, either to Josephine or to me, but I had, by then, attended enough people with terminal cancer to know that there was nothing more the hospital could offer her. However, my better judgement told me to wait until I was asked, before sharing that opinion.

'Will I get better?' Josephine asked me one day. It was the first time that I had had to see her in her bedroom, as she was too weak to get up and sit in the kitchen.

'Are you feeling any better?' I asked her, acknowledging, but not answering, her question, sitting down on the chair that her daughter had pulled up to her bedside, before she quietly slipped out of the room and left us alone.

'I don't know,' she replied. 'I was listening to the radio this morning and the music made me think I could dance, if I was just a little stronger.'

'I don't think you will dance again,' I said, looking directly at her. I didn't know how else to say it.

She looked surprised at first and then smiled gently, holding my gaze. 'No, I expect not,' she said. Looking down, she saw my hand resting on top of the pink, floral-patterned duvet cover and patted it gently. 'Thank you, Doctor,' she said.

I covered her hand with my own and remained silent.

Now, as I placed her file in the pile for archiving, I thought about the way I had developed an ease around caring for the dying that allowed me to provide not only good clinical care, but to respond to the needs of each individual and family. Because of my years of experience and practice, I could detect the first signs of frailty and could encourage individuals and families to be ready for what would inevitably follow. With the terminally ill, I could predict with greater accuracy how long it would be until the end. I had learned to work with the palliative care specialists and the Homecare team and used their services appropriately, but without abandoning the patients. The better I knew people, the more I could gauge how they and their families might cope with death and dying, even though I was wrong at times. Some families would surprise me with their ready acceptance, while others, who I thought would be well prepared, hid their fear and grief behind a fortress of denial.

With practice, I learned to manage my own emotions, leaving me with more to offer patients and their families. It wasn't that I did not feel sad or angry when yet another patient received a diagnosis of terminal disease, or didn't grieve when someone I cared for died. It wasn't that it did not remind me of my own mortality and cause me to question how I was spending my time. I was learning that these emotions and uncertainties were normal. I was no longer hiding from them or fighting them. I knew they would pass, and they did, without leaving me drained or overwhelmed. Sad, yes, but not despondent. Caring for the dying had taught me how to live. I had learned that those who embrace life can also embrace death. Their acceptance, appreciation and savouring of what was good eased their suffering. But those skills and attributes did not suddenly appear with the diagnosis of a terminal illness. They were habits that grew stronger with practice, day by day, a little at a time, a bit like my accordion playing.

CHAPTER EIGHTEEN

THE BARE NECESSITIES

Sorting files, keeping records, performing audits and managing emotions were just some of the behind-the-scenes challenges of running a successful GP practice. There were many other similar tasks and I had one in particular that I could not put off any longer. I needed a supply of ring pessaries for the older women patients who had uterine prolapse, and in order to get them, I had to pay a visit to the hospital stores to collect them.

For women who did not want, or could not have surgery, these pessaries were a safe and effective method of relieving symptoms, but to avoid complications, they had to be replaced every four months. Prior to my arrival in Killenaule, these women had attended the hospital gynaecology outpatient clinic three times a year for the procedure. There was no charge to the patient for that service, but most of them did not like going: there were often long delays in the clinic and they complained that they would meet a different doctor every time. Also, in the days of the Celtic Tiger, when everyone had employment, there was not always a family member available to drive them to the hospital and if they missed an appointment, they had to wait another few months for a further one. Therefore, it was good medical practice for me to do it and it was a procedure that was well within my competency. However, the only way I could get the pessaries was if I collected them myself. If I didn't, I could give the patient a prescription and they would have to buy them from the pharmacy. I figured that if the hospital could supply them for free, then I should be able to offer this also. The task of collecting the pessaries was far from straightforward, though, and each time I did it, I had to brace myself for the interrogation that I would have to endure before achieving my goal.

On that particular day, I drove to the hospital, parked in the car park and, with a heavy heart but steely determination, entered the building that housed the hospital supplies.

'Hello,' I called, as I pushed open the door to the large storeroom, my eyes searching for someone who looked as if they were in charge, or preferably someone who recognised me.

'Can I help you?' an unfamiliar man asked.

'I am Doctor Gannon,' I said, deliberately slowing my speech to counteract the tendency I have to talk too quickly when I am nervous, or when I anticipate a negative response. 'I have come to collect some supplies.'

The man looked me up and down, as if to say, 'You can't be much of a doctor, if this is what they have you doing. What department are you working in?' he asked.

This was exactly what I had been hoping to avoid. The interrogation had begun. 'I'm not in any department,' I replied. 'I am a GP in Killenaule.' I wasn't sure if the look he gave me was one of disregard or disbelief, if he had ever heard of Killenaule, or ever seen a GP here before, or if it was a mixture of both. I told myself I was being oversensitive and reoriented my attention to the task at hand.

'We don't normally give supplies to GPs,' he said. 'This is the hospital store. We only supply the hospital.'

I felt that he was telling me I had strayed too far out of my territory and I had better get back there, or anything could happen.

'I know,' I said. 'But a few years ago, I made a special arrangement with the Primary Care Unit manager and she contacted your store manager and both agreed that I could collect supplies from here.'

He wasn't convinced. 'I'll have to check that,' he said. 'I'll just go and see if I have any documentation to that effect. We have to account for everything here, so I can't just go giving stuff out without authorisation.'

'I don't think you will find any documentation,' I said. 'The man I met last time looked, but couldn't find any. I just signed for them and he said that should be OK.'

The man was walking away from me down an aisle between two rows of open shelving, stacked high with boxes and packages of all shapes and sizes. I could see the objects of my desire. I followed him down, trying to get his attention and save him a futile search. 'I made this arrangement a few years ago,' I repeated. 'I put in a proposal and asked if I could get supplies here for my patients. It's a cost-saving initiative for the hospital. They supply the tools, I do the work and patients don't have to go to the gynaecology clinic.'

My main problem was that since I had made the arrangement, the Primary Care Unit manager had moved to a more senior post, so it was unlikely that this man would find anybody who knew about our arrangement. We didn't think that it needed to be written down at the time. That was a big mistake.

The man appeared to have little interest in my explanation. We both stopped at a desk, cluttered with papers, dockets and half-empty boxes. He picked up what looked like a ledger, opened it and started to sift through the loose-leafed documents that had been stuck in at random between various pages. I tried not to look bored, frustrated, defensive or aggressive, although I was feeling a mixture of all four. I checked my body language, unfolded my arms, smiled and nodded at another man who happened to pass by with a handful of papers under his arm. I noticed we had a bit of an audience. The room had desks that looked like work stations, positioned at odd locations between the aisles. Some people stood at these desks looking in our direction, while others were coming and going with documents and papers, checking supplies and marking things down on their clipboards. There was a lot of activity in the storeroom and I noticed that all the workers were male.

I waited while my man checked through another heap of loose-leafed papers on the desk. He was wasting his time. Even if an authorisation document had been signed, it was unlikely to be sitting on that desk three years later and, even if by chance it was, he was never going to find it in that cluttered environment. I was growing impatient. I hummed a silent, tuneless mantra to keep myself from tapping my foot, re-folding my arms, sighing or huffing in frustration. The truth was that I had driven to the hospital to collect supplies for patients in order to save them the inconvenience of going to the hospital three times a year. I was not getting any additional payment for the service. I was not getting travel expenses and I was beginning to feel like I was doing something wrong. Like I was trying to get something for nothing. Like I was doing this for personal gain. Later, I would wonder why it is that we do not trust that people may have a natural disposition for benevolence, that we are so frequently suspicious of the motives of others. I was as guilty of this as anyone else. But at that time, I was not in reflective mode.

Calm down, I scolded myself. Just stay calm and you will be out of here before you know it. This man is just doing his job. He has no idea of the frustrations that you bring on yourself when you insist on doing things differently. No one asked you to do this. It was your own idea.

'I really don't think you will find an authorisation document.' I said, when I could no longer remain silent. 'I come in about twice a year and usually just sign a form. I have been doing it for at least three years.'

'Well, can you tell me when you were here last? I might find the form you signed then, and I will know what to give you.'

'I don't remember when I was here last,' I said, my voice beginning to rise in frustration and annoyance. 'And I don't get the same amount every time. I know what I need, and I know where they are and I usually do not have this much trouble getting them.'

I knew I had over-stepped the mark. He sensed my annoyance and took it personally. I had made it personal by implying that he was more awkward than the other people I had met. I had given him the upper hand.

'I'm just doing my job,' he said. 'Like I said, everything here has to be accounted for. I have never been asked for anything by a GP before, so I am just making sure that everything is above board.'

'I'm sorry,' I said. 'I didn't mean to imply that you were being deliberately unhelpful. I am not trying to get something for nothing. I am trying to improve the service to patients. But I understand that you have your job to do.'

'I'll have to check it with my boss,' he said then.

'Of course,' I replied. 'He will probably remember me.'

The man closed the ledger and looked up at me, making no move to contact anyone.

'I'll wait here,' I said, thinking that it would be best to remain in full view until I got what I wanted.

'Well, he's away today,' the man said. 'If you come back tomorrow, he will probably be here.'

He was really putting it up to me, but I was not going home without my supplies. I would use every resource I could think of to get them. I raised my voice, making sure I could be heard throughout the store. 'It's just some vaginal pessaries I am after,' I said, with an emphasis on the word *vaginal*. They are not for myself. I am not going to sell them or anything. I just have some women patients who ... '

He stopped in his tracks and came back towards me. The audience dispersed. It was as I had hoped. 'I'm sure when you explain to your boss that it is the GP who gets the ... '

He was, by that time, back at the desk. He produced a blank docket and handed it to me. 'Take whatever you want,' he said. 'Just write in whatever you have taken on this, sign it and leave it back on this desk.'

'Thank you so much,' I said, my mission almost accomplished. I took a large Dunnes Stores shopping bag from its hiding place in my handbag and took as many boxes of pessaries of varying sizes as would fit in it. I took so many that it was almost two years before I had to return. On my next trip, I boldly announced to the first person I met that I needed to replenish my supplies of vaginal ring pessaries. He didn't even ask me who I was.

Collecting supplies was only one example of the challenges of providing good clinical care. As our practice developed, it became evident that we were constantly struggling with dwindling resources. It seemed as if the more care we provided, the more we were expected to provide, but most of the time, greater workload did not attract additional resources. Our first ten years in Killenaule were years of growth and development. From 1996 until approximately 2006, government policies appeared to be committed to investment in general practice: GPs responded to this by improving their premises, expanding services and increasing quality of care. In our case, a greenfield site had been transformed into a thriving, vibrant GP surgery, with two doctors, two nurses, a secretary and a steady stream of GP registrars and medical students, who had experienced at first hand the rewards and challenges of being a rural doctor.

A significant proportion of this investment came from a complicated and bizarre scheme called the Indicative Drug Budgeting Scheme, the IDBS, which had been in existence since 1993. Under this scheme, GPs were allocated an annual indicative target for expenditure on drugs for GMS patients. Any general practitioner whose expenditure was less than the budget was allowed claim half of the 'savings' for investment in their practice. This money subsidised an extension to our surgery, computers, defibrillators, oxygen cylinders, ECG machines, warfarin-testing machines, minor surgery equipment and much more. This, in turn, translated into much-improved services for patients. The addition of a practice nurse to the team meant we were able to offer warfarin checks, diabetes checks and a cervical smear service long before national programmes were implemented; Liam's experience in rheumatology meant he could provide assessment and treatment of musculoskeletal problems, while my extended training in obstetrics and gynaecology gave me the expertise to provide a range of women's health services. Most of these were services that were not included in our GMS contract, but this did not matter as long as our overall income allowed us to cover our expenses and look after ourselves and our family.

Up until 2006, the future looked good for general practice. The knowledge, skills and attitudes of the younger doctors who came to work under our mentorship, who I met on Wednesdays in the GP Training Scheme, led me to believe that Ireland would have a steady supply of competent, compassionate doctors to take over when our generation retired. But I was wrong. From 2006, dark clouds began to gather over the landscape of general practice. 'GP' became synonymous with crisis and 'junior doctor' with emigration.

A well-known economist, Ludwig von Mises, once said, 'If the tailor goes to war against the baker, he must henceforth produce his bread for himself.' It appeared that the government had gone to war with GPs and it was getting harder and harder for us to 'produce the bread'. It was not the policy makers or the government who were the victims of this war, but the most vulnerable in society, the people who needed complex, continuous primary care. The IDBS was abruptly withdrawn in 2006. Also around that time, payments to GPs for providing women's health clinics were discontinued. Annual fees for looking after elderly patients were reduced.

As the 2008 global recession progressed, the Financial Emergency Measures in the Public Interest (FEMPI) cuts resulted in the abolition of 'distance-codes' payments for GPs, a measure that had significantly reduced the payments received for rural patients living at a distance from the surgery. In the following years, all fees and allowances for both patients and staff were reduced, so that by the time of the fourth and final FEMPI cut in 2013, GPs had experienced a 38 per cent reduction in pre-expenses income, much more than politicians or any other public servants. Despite the fact that these were meant to be emergency measures, they have yet to be reversed. Alongside this reduction in income, the demand for free GP services was increasing, as was the complexity of the diseases being treated and the expectation that GPs take on more and more responsibility for chronic disease management.

Not long ago, I read an analysis of the reasons for the collapse of the road bridge in Genoa in August 2018. The author stated that the bridge did not have enough structural redundancies, so that when one cable gave way, the whole bridge collapsed. It struck me that general practice, like the bridge, has no structural redundancies. These have been deliberately removed, causing the structure to grow weaker under the ever-increasing traffic, leaving it in danger of complete collapse.

As long ago as the eighteenth century, Adam Smith recognised that 'it is not from the benevolence of the butcher, the brewer or the baker that we expect our dinner, but from their regard to their own interest'. Most GPs I know are a healthy mixture of benevolence and self-interest. When what we do helps us look after ourselves and our families, we do that work well and everybody is a winner. Any threat to our livelihood leads to one of three things: fight, flight or freeze. Following the fourth FEMPI cut to Irish GPs in 2013, GPs all across the country were choosing their response.

It was inevitable that the GPs' response would affect the doctor–patient relationship. One of my first experiences of this was with Imelda, a middle-aged patient who until then had never complained or indicated that she was in any way dissatisfied with the service that she received. One Monday morning, however, she bustled into my consulting room and slapped a document on my desk, pushing it towards me in an angry and determined manner.

I was caught unawares and invited her to sit down so that I could read it and see what was troubling her. She sat tersely on the edge of the chair. 'It is a letter from the HSE,' she said. 'It says in it that you have to do my blood tests and that you cannot charge me for them. In fact, you have to give me back the money I paid you last month for taking my bloods.'

I wasn't expecting that. Liam and I had decided a few months earlier that we would charge for blood tests, a service that we had provided free of charge until then. It was not a decision that had been taken lightly. I did not wish to upset any of my patients, but I could not sit back while government policies threatened my livelihood and made it very unlikely that newly qualified young GPs would take on GMS lists, or even set up in private practice in Ireland. (Purely private practice is no longer an appealing option anywhere in Ireland, as over 50 per cent of the population is currently entitled to free GP care, so most practices are a mixture of both private and public patients.) Charging for blood tests was not just about the money: it was a statement that from then on, Liam and I would work as close as possible to our contract and, after close examination of that same contract, we decided that it did not include routine phlebotomy services. All patients had been advised of the change of practice and offered referral to the hospital for blood tests, if they did not wish to pay for them. Those who chose to have them done in the surgery had been asked to sign a consent form to confirm that they had been made aware of the charge and were prepared to pay it. This included Imelda.

I explained once again to Imelda that she had been offered this choice and had chosen to avail of our service. I had not tricked her or forced her and while I was sorry that she was upset about it, there was nothing more I could do. I picked up the document that Imelda had pushed towards me, and glanced at it briefly before handing it back to her. She looked small and dejected, but was no longer angry. I sat back in my chair, relaxed my shoulders, which I realised had been up around my ears since she had come in and addressed her in a much softer tone. 'I am really sorry to have to charge you for something that was free up until now,' I said. 'And I can understand why you are upset and why you have reported this to the HSE. I would probably have done the same myself, if I was in your situation.'

She did not respond, just sat with her head lowered, the document still in her hand. I continued, 'I understand that you must be worried that the service you have been getting here is going to come to an end. You are right to be concerned. I am also fearful that when I leave, there will not be a doctor to replace me. But this is exactly why we have decided to charge for this particular service. Even though all our fees and allowances have been cut, we still have to pay the nurse to take the bloods and all the costs of keeping this place open. It is because we want to stay here that we made that decision. I don't know how else to explain it, except to say that you and I want the same things: a good-quality medical service for the people of Killenaule and other rural dwellers around the country. We should not be fighting each other. I don't blame you for being angry. I will continue to provide the best care I can with the resources I have, as I have always done.'

It was quite a long spiel and I am not sure if I was saying it for my own or for Imelda's benefit, but I felt better when I had spoken.

Imelda put the letter in her bag. 'I didn't realise that things had got so bad for GPs,' she said. 'I didn't mind paying, but I was worried that that might be just the start of it and that I might have to start paying for visits next. There's been a lot of talk about the charge for blood tests and I suppose, like you, I just didn't want to let it go without challenging it. But thank you for explaining things. It's a relief to know that it is only the bloods we have to pay for.'

With that, she left and I heaved a sigh of relief. My morning's work was far from over, but my resolve to continue to serve this community by whatever means necessary was strengthened. I could not expect my patients to understand the effects of government policies on general practice. As far as they were concerned, very little had changed for them, but we were working harder and doing longer hours than ever, our staff had endured pay cuts and our premises and equipment were badly in need of repair and replacement, if we were to continue to provide good-quality care. It is a testament to the resilience, business acumen and creativity of GPs that so many of us have survived the recession and are still in business. Sadly, even this has not been enough to prevent others from closing their businesses, leaving many patients without a GP.

CHAPTER NINETEEN

PRACTICE MAKES PERFECT

One morning in 2012, I lay awake, waiting for the clock to show six o'clock. As yet, there was no sound from the rest of the house. I was waiting for Ailshe to come and wake me, when I would pretend that I had been asleep all along, with no worries about the events of the day to come. When she did, we would climb the little staircase to the attic room where I kept my computer, to check her Health Professions Admission Test (HPAT) results. She did not feel capable of doing this herself. In a short time, she would know whether or not six years of studying, memorising, revising, problem-solving, analysing, time-managing and, most important, strategic planning, had paid off. In a short time, she would know if she could plan her departure from school, home and Killenaule to enter one of the country's medical schools. The result of the test would decide her fate.

Ailshe had wanted to be a doctor since she was little. She had watched every episode of *Gray's Anatomy* at least ten times. By the age of fifteen, she could name the small bones of the hand, list the symptoms of diabetes, check a pulse and use a stethoscope as well as any final-year medical student. However, she might as well have had a special talent for growing geraniums or identifying ancient fossils for all the good this would do her in securing a place in medicine.

The Health Professions Admission Test was introduced in 2009 as a means of widening access to medical schools, which, until then, had welcomed only the the top achievers in the Leaving Cert examination. The new examination, the HPAT, had four distinct sections, which claimed to measure logical reasoning, problem-solving, non-verbal reasoning and the ability to understand the thoughts and behaviours of others. It was a three-hour examination that demanded extreme levels of concentration. The strict time limit meant that many candidates did not manage to complete it. A high score in this test with a relatively good Leaving Certificate would guarantee a place in medicine. A low score meant that a place was highly unlikely, regardless of Leaving Certificate points.

When the HPAT was first introduced, students were told that there was no point trying to prepare for the examination. It was not possible to improve your scores. You either had the personality traits and attributes that made you a good doctor, or you didn't. Popular media also hinted that boys were more likely to do well in the test than girls. This was subsequently found to be correct, with boys scoring consistently higher in three of the four categories. In the 'ability to understand the thoughts and behaviours of others', girls score higher. With my ever-present sense of unease about the undermining of women, I wondered if indeed the test had actually been introduced to correct the fact that more girls were entering medicine at that time than boys. Liam dismissed this as paranoia.

Despite this perceived bias, or perhaps because of it, young women all over the country took up the challenge of attaining maximum points in the Leaving Cert, maximum points in the HPAT and marched onwards towards their destination. Likewise, young women and men also chose to disregard the advice that there was no point preparing for the HPAT. Those who could afford it signed up for one of the many HPAT preparatory courses that had sprung up around the country, promising what had been previously deemed impossible: preparation for the test with guaranteed improvement in scores. There was nothing like saying something could not be done to make these determined and motivated young people want to prove it could. So, amidst all this uncertainty, not quite sure what to believe and with no way of knowing if it was the right thing to do, in the October of her Leaving Cert year, when she should have been taking a mid-term break, Ailshe booked an HPAT preparatory course.

When I went to meet her at the end of her first day she was almost in tears. 'It's just awful, Mum,' she said. 'Most of the people in there already have six hundred points in their Leaving Cert and are spending this year just studying for the HPAT. And I can't answer any of the questions. It's impossible to know what answer they want. I don't understand it, even *after* it's been explained to me. I don't get it. I'm just not good enough.'

I had never heard her like that before. There was nothing I could say. Perhaps those who said you either 'had it or you hadn't' were right. Perhaps there was no point preparing. I had looked at a sample paper and even with years of practical experience, I had no idea why one answer was right and another wrong. Suddenly, I became aware of my thought processes. I was beginning to believe the nonsense. Beginning to doubt Ailshe's ability. Of course, there was no way she was not good enough. There is no such thing as 'not good enough'. How can any test decide whether or not an 18-year-old would make a 'good' doctor? No one is born with the necessary attributes to be a doctor. No one has such a fixed personality that they can not improve on some attributes. Everything can be improved with practice. Language, maths, skiing, running, piano, listening and communication skills, gratitude and compassion. Wasn't this what I was trying to convey to the GP registrars in our Wednesday workshops? Anything could be improved with practice.

I did not share these thoughts with Ailshe. She was too overwrought, too disappointed, too influenced by the collective subconscious to be interested in my analysis. Besides, I had not had to sit a HPAT. I had not even had to decide to do medicine. I just had to go about happily doing whatever subjects I wanted to for Leaving Cert and at the end of it be offered a place, if I wanted it. I was quite sure no test would have singled me out at the age of 18 as a potential 'good' doctor. Also, I didn't know what it was like to work almost six years for something, only to begin to believe that it was beyond my grasp.

So I kept quiet for the moment and suggested we go to Fat Freddy's on Quay Street for pizza. It felt good to be in a Galway restaurant on a weekday evening, a place that did not exist when I was a student there and even if it did, I would not have been able to afford to eat there. So it felt good to be there, to be able to afford to eat out, to be able to afford the HPAT course and to be able to take time off from my work to accompany Ailshe to Galway to attend it. This was what I was most glad of. That I was there and that at least she could tell me how she felt. I was witness to her disappointment but could temper it. Because even though I may not have had to dedicate six years to getting into medicine and had not had to sit an HPAT examination, I had been a doctor for many years and I knew that Ailshe was 'good enough' to be one, too. She was bright, motivated and empathetic. She would try her best at whatever job she did and she would do it well.

I turned my attention back to my surroundings, allowing the hum of conversation, the flickering candlelight, the eclectic mix of wall-hangings and memorabilia, and the pizza, to soothe us both and to restore a sense of equilibrium. Potential diners entered the restaurant, their eyes gradually adjusting to the light, automatically assessing the ambience and busyness of the place. Others got up, paid their bills, pulled on raincoats and hats as protection against the rain that seemed to be for ever falling in Galway, and left.

Little by little, I sensed the opening of a space for perspective. I decided to go there and try to expand it. I asked Ailshe if she remembered the day when she was around eight and had just started to learn the piano. 'Do you remember, we were in the music shop in Kilkenny and you picked up the sheet music to "Bohemian Rhapsody"?'

She nodded.

'And you said that it looked so difficult and that you could never imagine being able to play it.'

'And it wasn't long before I could,' she said. 'I know what you are saying, Mum. If I give up now, then I will never know if I could have achieved a good-enough result.'

She decided that she would see how she felt by the end of the course and re-evaluate her options then. We left it at that. The only way to eat that elephant was one bite at a time.

Lying awake in bed on the morning of the results, I remembered that by day three of the course, Ailshe's attitude had changed. It was as if a different girl emerged. A girl with a plan, because even by day three, her scores on the practice exams had started to improve. It was the same for everybody else, she said. And that was all the encouragement that was needed. For the rest of the year, she did practice exams against the clock for half an hour every evening, as part of her homework. Week on week, her scores improved, so that when the time came to sit the examination that February, she was feeling very confident of an adequate score. All the background noise of it not being possible to prepare and of having a better chance if you were male, had long since been assigned to the 'making no sense' area of the brain. It was time to see if her efforts had paid off.

'Mum,' she shook me gently, even though my eyes were wide open. 'It's six o'clock.'

'I know,' I said getting out of bed. 'How did you sleep?'

'Surprisingly well,' she said. 'I only woke with the alarm.'

We climbed the stairs in silence. I sat at the desk in front of the computer, pressed the button and waited for the screen to light up. Ailshe sat on the two-seater couch that was positioned under the 'spy' window, the skylight through which, years earlier, her brothers had imagined shooting arrows at unwelcome visitors. She held the instructions for the website in her hand. She was folded in on herself, holding the paper in front of her, and with minimum movement, read out the steps slowly and deliberately: website address, username, password, exam results. I followed them all, breathing deeply to slow my pounding heart. The result of this exam would determine her immediate future. It wasn't life or death. It wasn't like it was the result of a biopsy or an MRI scan, but for an eighteen-year-old who had spent the last six years working towards a specific goal, who was one hundred per cent sure that this is what she wanted to do with her life, who had given it her very best effort, this was a significant moment.

I scrolled down the alphabet until I got to M. 'OK,' I said. 'I'm scrolling.'

Ailshe had unfurled herself a little and was sitting with her head in her hands, the instructions bunched up tightly in her fist. I wondered what was going through her head. I kept talking. 'It looks like the results are displayed right across from the names, so when I click on Meagher, I will see your result straight away and call it out. I'm at Meagher,' I said. 'Will I click?'

'Just a minute,' she said.

I took my fingers off the keyboard and sat back, looking away from her, allowing her to gather herself, to perhaps go through the two scenarios in her head and prepare a reaction.

'OK, I'm ready,' she said.

I leaned forward, placing my fingers over the keyboard once again.

'Well, no. Wait. Just another minute.' She closed her eyes, took a deep breath in and slowly exhaled, opened her eyes and said, 'OK, you can go ahead. Just say my name first and then give me a second before the result.'

'Ailshe Meagher,' I said and paused, as she had asked me to.

'Oh, Mum, just tell me,' she said, almost in tears. 'I can take it, if it's not good.'

'OK, here goes.' I checked again to make sure I had the right name and number, even though I knew it had to be, as I would not have had access to any other result. I called out her score. She looked at me, wide-eyed, and if she had not been sitting down, I am quite sure she would have fainted.

'You are well clear of that hurdle anyway,' I said, smiling, feeling happy and relieved.

Tears of joy and relief were flowing unchecked down her face.

I went to sit beside her and give her a hug. 'Well done.' I said. 'Very well deserved.'

'You're sure you got the right results, Mum?' she said.

'One hundred per cent sure,' I replied.

She didn't have the energy to check. She took my word for it for once. Even though it would be another couple of months before her Leaving Cert results would be available, she knew that unless something completely bizarre were to happen, she was almost certainly going to be offered a place in a medical school. The following September, she would enter another phase of her life as a medical student. I was quite sure that she would have a very different experience from that of both Liam and me: students and registrars had told me that the rules and regulations had tightened up significantly since my time, with daily signing-in to tutorials and lectures in some colleges. Gone were the days when simply passing the exam was enough. However, I was also confident that she was more than ready to embark on this new adventure.

Alongside those of my own children, I could not help but have an interest in the Leaving Certificate results of my younger patients. Sixth year was a stressful year and I always checked with this age group if they were in an exam year, as very often this might explain why they increased their consultation rates. Miranda was one such person. A few weeks after the Leaving Certificate results, Miranda came in to have a contraceptive implant procedure, and as she sat in front of me, her face a picture of satisfaction and optimism, I knew before she spoke that she had achieved her goal. As usual, I waited for her to tell me in her own time, in case I was mistaken and the news was not good.

'I got my course,' Miranda announced, with a smile.

'That's fantastic,' I replied. 'So, you'll be off to Maynooth in September.'

'Yep, I can't wait.'

It was great to see Miranda in such good form. During her Leaving Cert year, exam pressure had robbed her temporarily of her sleep, her appetite, her characteristic optimism and her cheerfulness. If she had been in paid employment, I would have recommended that she take time off to rest and relax, but there was no taking time off from the final-year exams. The year always marched on with the certainty of the seasons, starting in September with homework, revision and weekend grinds. Mock examinations were the focus for spring, followed by oral and practical exams and ending with written exams in the summer.

Now, all of that was behind her. Miranda had achieved her goal and could look forward to a new phase of her life, away from home, school, and Killenaule.

I was happy for her because this was what she wanted, not because I thought this was what everyone her age should do. There were other young people who chose not to go to college or university, whose school experiences had not been positive and who never wanted to look at another book or sit another exam again. I felt just as happy for them when they told me about their new job, new car, or new relationship. However, being the mother of two Leaving Cert students – Joseph, having completed his Leaving Cert a couple of years earlier, was studying finance and economics at University College Dublin – with another one to go, had given me insight into the highs and lows of the education system and the angst associated with exams, the choosing of colleges and the carving of career paths.

'How did the maths go?' I asked Miranda.

'I got a B1,' she said. 'I'm delighted.' Miranda had considered moving from the honours to the pass maths class as she was convinced that she was not fit for honours, but her teacher had persuaded her not to do this.

'So your teacher was right,' I said. As I was prepping her arm and preparing the anaesthetic, I kept talking to her in order to distract her, as she appeared a little anxious about the procedure. I felt a bit ancient as I rambled on about how in my day, girls were not encouraged to do honours maths. That it was considered a subject more suitable for engineers and architects and other male occupations. That was a long time ago: girls were now competing with boys for all of these occupations and were performing just as well, if not better, in subjects like honours maths, physics and technical graphics. But with these opportunities came responsibility and challenge. I had previously read articles in the popular press expressing the view that girls were wasting these opportunities, that they were taking up valuable places on courses and would never contribute the equivalent of their male counterparts to the workforce. That they would qualify and quit, go on to have babies and squander their qualifications and training. I had heard this view expressed publicly and privately in medical circles, where the term 'feminisation of medicine' had become synonymous with the undermining of the profession by women, who only wanted to work part-time or take time off for childcare.

Liam told me I was being hypersensitive and paranoid when I voiced this opinion, or tried to explain my unease. As a man who advocated equal opportunity for all, who believed that parental leave should be available to fathers or mothers, depending on a particular family's situation, who shared household responsibilities and childcare, he did not understand how anyone could think that a woman was less valuable than a man in the workplace, any more than believing a man was less valuable than a woman in the home. However, he read the sports and politics sections of the newspaper, while I preferred the opinion editorials, and so we had different views of the world.

I did not worry about this attitude for myself, as I was already well established in my career, but I feared that it undermined young women, like Ailshe and Miranda, who were embarking on careers and who needed encouragement, rather than disapproval and scepticism. I did not share this with Miranda and before long the procedure was completed, the arm was bandaged and I was sending her on her way with instructions to avoid washing windows, hoovering floors or lifting heavy shopping bags for at least six months.

It took her a second to realise I wasn't serious. 'Not that I have any plans for washing windows anytime soon,' she said, as she hopped off the couch and grabbed her jacket from the hook, anxious to get away and get on with the rest of her day.

I felt a familiar pang when saying goodbye. It was always a bittersweet experience when young people gained entry to college and set out on the next part of their life's journey. Just as I had to let my own children go, I had to let these young patients go. It was unlikely that I would ever be Miranda's main carer again.

'If I don't see you before you go, I wish you the very best of luck,' I said to Miranda. 'Look after yourself and you know where I am if you ever need me. I'll probably be here for another few years anyway, so I should be around to replace that implant when it needs to be done. But be sure and link in with the college medical services. You are far better off with a doctor on site if you need one.'

'Thanks, Doctor. I will,' she said.

She was gone without a backward glance. It was as it should be. I made my note and closed her file. My next appointment was already waiting, a young mother with her new baby attending for a two-week check.

'Congratulations,' I said to the mother when she was settled in the chair, the baby still asleep in a car seat that looked like a miniature sleeping pod in a Google office.

'Thank you, Doctor,' she replied, beaming.

As we both admired the sleeping baby, I couldn't help but wonder if there would be anyone sitting in my chair when this little one came to do her Leaving Cert. If she would have anyone to consult when she felt exam pressure, anyone to provide a contraceptive implant or to feel a tinge of sadness as she left Killenaule and moved into the wider world.

A BAD PATIENT

I sat, head bent, in the waiting room of the private hospital, trying to concentrate on the book I had taken from the small library beside the reception window. It was a book of essays written by a doctor, but I wasn't really reading it. I was waiting for my sister Marian to join me, and each time I heard footsteps approaching, or the gentle opening of the door, I looked up to see if it was her, immediately redirecting my gaze to the book when it wasn't. She wasn't late; I was early.

The waiting room was quiet and calm and if it weren't for the repeated ringing of the telephone and the voice of the receptionist answering it, I could have imagined I was in a spa, awaiting a rejuvenating foot treatment or an Indian head massage. To get to this inner sanctum, I had come through a large foyer and advanced up the wide curved staircase to the first floor, past the busy cafeteria, where people in scrubs sat with people in nurses' uniforms and other people in normal clothes, who, I assumed, were patients or relatives. No one but staff, patients or relatives would choose to eat in a hospital cafeteria on a Wednesday afternoon in January.

I rested the book on my lap and looked around me for the first time since I had come in. A lady in a wheelchair sat opposite me, accompanied by a man, who, I presumed, was her husband – I was making lots of presumptions about people that day. They were talking in hushed tones, in keeping with the general ambience of the place. An elegant-looking older woman, probably in her early seventies, sat a few chairs away. She had smiled at me when I came in and I had returned her smile with a polite, reserved one that was not meant to encourage conversation. She had obviously not picked up on this cue because, before long, she addressed me. 'Who are you for?' she asked in a normal tone of voice, but which sounded inappropriately loud in that setting.

I reluctantly told her which consultant I was waiting for, before returning to my book. I really did not want to engage her in conversation, but she seemed keen, so I relented. I wasn't really able to concentrate on the book anyway and perhaps she was just anxious about her appointment and needed some idle conversation to keep her mind off it. 'Have you been waiting long?' I asked, thinking that if I was going to have a conversation, I might as well take charge of it and steer it in a direction of my choosing. As I got older, I found I was more likely to engage with strangers, but also more adept at not giving away too much information.

'Oh, no,' she replied. 'You never have to wait long here. Not like the public hospitals. I used to spend all day waiting for clinic appointments there.'

'Hmm, I know what you mean,' I replied. My main experience of public hospitals had been sitting in emergency departments with my injured children. During those long waits, I would often feel like rolling up my sleeves and offering my services. It wasn't that I was really keen for work; it was just that I would have done anything to shorten the wait.

Silence once again descended on the room and I thought about resuming my reading. Was there a waiting room etiquette?

I wondered. How much engagement was expected? Was there a normal range? It wasn't unusual for Annemarie, our latest secretary, to appear at my side in the middle of a surgery, asking me to please call a garrulous or gossipy patient in ahead of their turn, as they were making the more reserved types uncomfortable. My elegant companion-in-waiting was not garrulous, but neither was she reserved. Just when I had resolved to return to my book, I heard her speak again.

'Is it arthritis you have?' she asked. 'You don't look like someone with arthritis. You look like you don't have a thing wrong with you.'

I was taken aback by the directness of her question, by the loudness of her voice. It felt almost like a physical assault and I am sure I flinched. I found it difficult to disguise my irritation, my distaste for her invasion of my privacy. The man and woman sitting opposite me looked at me, but looked away again quickly, as if they were embarrassed by the lady's question and wanted to distance themselves from it. The woman asked the man to get her a tissue from her bag. I knew that I wasn't the only one who felt that this was a breach of etiquette.

To cover my discomfiture, I gave a nervous laugh and asked just as audibly, 'What does someone with arthritis look like? I didn't know it was that easy to tell.'

Before she could answer, the door opened and my sister rushed in, apologising for being late and blaming the afternoon traffic and the difficulty getting parked. The lady smiled at Marian and left us to ourselves, as we chatted in hushed spa tones.

In contrast to the waiting area, the consultant's room was large, bright and cheerful, with a window stretching the full length of one wall and an impressive array of computer screens on the large spacious work space. This was a digital doctor, clearly. Patient files, MRI scans and treatment protocols were all neatly tucked away in the computer software system, but still easily accessible at the touch of a keyboard. It was this consultant's online presence that had led me to his consulting room on that day in 2013. Unbeknownst to him, he had been my Twitter role model when I had taken my first tentative steps onto that online platform a few years earlier, someone who was a good few steps ahead and whose online presence exuded professionalism and compassion. I felt sure that this would be the case in the real, as well as the virtual, world.

I introduced him to my sister, before taking my seat. He smiled, took her hand and gave her a welcoming handshake. All three of us sat down. He did not shake my hand, nor did I expect him to. We had gone to the same university and had attended the same rheumatology tutorials. I remembered little from those tutorials, as I was usually so terrified that I would be asked a question and would not be able to answer that my higher cognitive function shut down and I spent the whole of the class in a state of fight or flight. But I did remember being taught not to squeeze the hand of a patient with rheumatoid arthritis, because it could possibly hurt them. I knew this and had always observed it myself, but I was not prepared for the feeling that the omission of that universal gesture of connection engendered in me. I felt that I had been singled out, that I was no longer inhabiting the land of the healthy. It did not matter how well I looked, or what image I portrayed to the world: I was in this consulting room because I was a patient. A patient with a chronic disease that would be with me for the rest of my life and would need treatment and monitoring.

Of course, I had known this a few weeks earlier. I had known it as I drove to the specialist's appointment that day. Every morning, I knew it when I woke and moved slowly about the bedroom waiting for my joints to lose their stiffness, from the pain I felt in my hands as I squeezed the bulb of the sphygmomanometer when measuring patients' blood pressure. I knew it when my feet touched the ground and I felt as if I was walking on marbles, or when I felt the late-afternoon fatigue that I continuously fought to overcome. I knew it, but I never really felt it until that day, when, out of kindness and a wish not to inflict pain, another person did not shake my hand. Which was worse? I wondered later. The momentary, unintentional pain engendered by another person's hand squeezing yours, or the realisation that you now inhabit a place slightly outside the social norms, a place that I had once heard described by Susan Sontag as 'the kingdom of the sick'?

I wish I could say that the events that resulted in my presenting myself as a patient to the rheumatologist at that moment had begun a few weeks, or months, or even years earlier. That would imply that I knew the exact moment that my body had started to malfunction. But transitioning from health to disease is like going from the past to the present. Where does one end and the other begin? There is no defining divide. All we can say about disease is that at some point we become aware of it. It gets to a point where we cannot ignore it. Diseases like diabetes, heart disease and rheumatoid arthritis are written in the blueprint of some and not others. Like soldiers on a secret mission, they start their slow march under cover of darkness and attack when the circumstances are favourable, or when provoked.

I am not sure why my particular army of soldiers attacked about three months prior to my rheumatology appointment. Their first target was my knee. They then moved to my shoulder on their way to the small joints of my hands and feet, where they engaged in a more persistent battle. Meanwhile, I kept doing what I was doing, going to work, going to the cinema, and meeting Judith for our usual walks. I diagnosed myself with post-viral arthralgia, a swelling in the joints that can come after a virus (even though I had not had a virus), fibromyalgia, a debilitating muscular condition, but one that did not result in joint damage if untreated (even though I knew this was definitely not a likely explanation) and in the evenings, when the pain and stiffness had subsided, I even convinced myself that it was nothing at all, imagining that if I ignored it, I would wake one morning and feel well again.

Until one day, when Judith rang. I answered her from the couch, where I had been lying since leaving the shopping on the kitchen table a couple of hours earlier. 'I'm sorry,' I said. 'Not today. I cannot go out for a walk today.'

Later, when Liam came in and found me still in the same position, he laid his hand on mine and repeated what he had been saying for weeks. 'Lucia, we both know what you have. Are you ready to at least let me do your bloods, or go and get someone else to do it?'

I did have a GP, but I rarely went to see her. The previous time I attended her, she'd asked me if she was still my GP, as it was so long since she had seen me. I did not like going to doctors. I was not a 'good' patient. I did not like to bother her. I knew how busy she was. The rare time I did go, I would offer my diagnosis and a ready-made plan, rather than my symptoms. I did not like to be a burden. I told myself that I did not want any doctor charged with the cognitive load of figuring out what to do for me. That may have been true, but I also think that I did not like to hand over control, to let go of the reins and maybe, just maybe, there was a little bit of me that believed I knew best and I did not trust another GP to make a plan for me. Whatever, the reasons, I was not one for seeing my GP. I did not have this difficulty consulting a specialist. They had been specially trained. They were supposed to know more than me on a particular topic. With a specialist, it was much easier for me to get out of the driving seat.

I was done with resisting. I had reached acceptance, the first step on the road to a different way of being. I was both doctor and patient and I knew what lay ahead. There was no other way except forward. I would accept the diagnosis, take the medication and be glad that I could. On a rational level, I knew that there were much worse diseases than rheumatoid arthritis. I knew I was lucky to live in an era when there was access to effective treatments. But throughout all my years of practice, I had never forgotten a frail little old lady whom I used to visit as a GP registrar in Sudbury, Derbyshire. Her slight frame was permanently stooped and rigid. Her joints creaked as she moved slowly ahead of me from the front door to the sitting room. Her hands, like little bags of thinly covered bones, were contorted into the classical 'rheumatoid' shapes, no longer painful, but stiff and rigid. At the time that she was diagnosed, the only treatment available would have been anti-inflammatory medication, which did nothing to prevent joint damage. Hers was the image that always came to mind when I thought of rheumatoid arthritis. Even though I frequently reassured the patients I cared for that they would not end up with contorted and twisted fingers and wrists, I had not believed my own words and despite all my medical training, I was a likely as anyone else to be haunted by the ghosts of diseases past.

I left the consultant's office with a plan, a prescription and a sense of perspective. I was active and otherwise healthy and there was no reason to think that this should alter my life in any way, once I stuck to that plan and paid attention to getting enough exercise and rest.

Three months later, I wrestled my ringing phone from the pocket of my rain jacket, swiped the screen and managed with difficulty to put it to my ear, which was well covered with a hat and a hood. I turned my back to the wind and the rain that had just started to fall. It was my mother. 'Where are you?' she asked. 'It sounds like there's a gale blowing wherever you are.'

'You could say that,' I replied. 'I'm at the top of Slievenamon. I should be looking out at the Galtees, but I can't see anything except clouds and mist and if I don't get down from here soon, I'll definitely be blown away.'

'Good God, Lucia,' she said. 'What are you doing up there? Should you not be resting yourself?' I might be a doctor, but that never stopped my mother giving me medical advice, or updating me on newspaper articles or television documentaries that purported to have found the latest treatments for all manner of diseases.

'Could you not have waited for a good day at least?' she asked then.

'It is a good day,' I replied. 'You know what they say here. Any day you are above ground …'

'Well, I was just thinking of you,' she said, 'and wanted to see if you were OK.'

I reassured her that I was well and happy and was not doing myself any harm by getting out and about. She reluctantly accepted that I might know what I was talking about. I replaced my phone in my pocket, faced into the wind and quickened my step to catch up with Judith, who was already almost half-way down the mountain. My mother was right. It probably would have been better to wait for a 'good day,' but as I got older, I was beginning to realise that life was too short and too unpredictable to wait too long.

CHAPTER TWENTY-ONE

BACK ON TRACK

It was a Monday morning and I was almost half-way through the morning surgery. All of my ten-minute appointment slots were filled with mostly familiar names, in an ordered line beneath my name. This did not mean that I would see them in an orderly fashion. Some patients came late: they might have had an unexpected delay at the school gate, or a phone call from a daughter in Australia, just as they were going out of the door. More often than not, it was me who was responsible for the delay. Despite years of consulting, I had not yet mastered the art of consistently taking a history, performing an examination and forming a plan in ten minutes. I could do it for some, but not for everyone. Nonetheless, booking people in every ten minutes was the best way for me to manage my day. Neither I nor the patient could say how long we would need. We did the best we could and I usually managed to finish in a reasonable time.

That day, up until that point I was the epitome of efficiency and I was happy. I congratulated myself on this little success, finished the note on the patient I had just seen, skipped out to the waiting room and called, 'Philip O'Shea, please'.

Philip rose and came towards me. Holding the door to my consulting room open, I smiled as I waited for him to come in and take a seat. He took his place, as he had done so many times before, in the empty chair, placed at an angle to mine, only the curved edge of my desk separating them. Immediately, I checked my high spirits, because something in the way he had entered the room, not greeting me or returning my smile, alerted me to a need for something other than efficiency: a seriousness, a slowing down.

As he sat, he moved the chair back slightly from the desk. I wasn't sure if this was accidental, or if it meant that he was undecided as to how much he was going to share with me that day. I waited. He kept his head bowed, avoiding eye contact, hands immobile on his lap. A man in his early sixties, Philip was wearing Nike tracksuit bottoms and runners with a light puffa jacket over a white T-shirt. His face was clean-shaven and he had a full head of greying hair, neatly cut, in a style younger than his years. He began to unzip the jacket, still not speaking. I waited another couple of seconds as he struggled with how to begin. Sitting forward, I moved my chair a little to angle it away from my computer so that I was facing him. Conscious that he might want to maintain some distance, but keen to indicate my willingness to connect, I sat forward, elbows resting on the desk and wordlessly invited him to begin. Finally, he looked up at me, with no words for his feelings, and I knew I would have to help him.

'How are you today, Philip?' I asked, my tone sombre and serious. It was my usual opening gambit when people were struggling for words, something I had learned from a depressed young woman when I'd worked as a junior doctor in psychiatry. 'Sometimes, today is the only day I can think about,' she had said. 'If you have to ask me how I am, ask me only about today.'

Philip looked up and held my gaze. 'Would you believe, today is not a bad day,' he said. 'I have had some very bad days, but at least today, I got out of bed and came over here.' I remained silent.

Now that he had started, he would be best left to tell me his story in his own words, in his own time and without my prompting. 'It's not getting any easier,' he went on after a short pause, 'I miss her so much and still can't believe that she is gone.'

I remained silent. It had been three months since Philip's wife had died and I had seen him a couple of times since then. He had been managing as expected but that day I sensed a difference, an overwhelming despondency that he needed to share. I would serve him best by listening.

Philip cleared his throat and sighed deeply, before continuing. 'Last Wednesday I drove to the train station,' he said. 'I had no plan to go anywhere and sort of ended up on the platform. I was millimetres from the edge and I could hear the train coming. I thought how easy it would be to jump. I looked around to see if there was anyone there to push me. I would have given anything for someone to push me in front of that train. I stood there and willed myself to fall forward. It should have been so easy. I should have been able to just let myself go. But I just couldn't do it.' He looked up but quickly turned away again.

I sat immobile, without speaking, allowing the gravity of his words to sink in, trying to imagine what it must be like for him to stand on a platform, hoping that that the end would come, that in an instant he would be released from this life, that the vast expanse of nothingness after death was better than what he had to endure every day.

After a few seconds he resumed his story. 'There were people on the platform, but no one was paying any attention to me. It would have been so easy to just do it. But I couldn't. It was a very bad day, Doctor. I thought I'd better come and talk to you.'

I glimpsed a tiny ray of hope. A hand outstretched from the turbulent ocean of grief. 'Why could you not do it?' I asked. 'What stopped you?' I was trying to connect with the part of him that had chosen to live. The part of him that might grab a lifebuoy that could keep him afloat until he could swim unaided.

'I was too afraid,' was his reply. 'At the last minute, I just couldn't let myself go.'

I waited to see if he wanted to say more, but he remained silent, head still bowed, resting in the silence after the effort of speaking.

'How do you feel now?' I asked. Are you glad you didn't succeed?'

I couldn't say the word 'jump'. It was too vivid. Too evocative. He didn't reply, so I asked an easier question, to help him speak again. 'What did you do, afterwards, once the train had pulled away?'

'I think I just came home,' he replied. 'I don't really remember driving back, but I must have come back. I remember when I got home, I felt a bit angry with myself at first, but then I felt relieved.'

I assumed it was relief that he was still alive, but after a short pause he went on. 'I know now that at least there is a way out, if I really can't bear it. I know I can do it, if I really need to. That is what gets me through the day now, Doctor. I know that's not right, but it gets me through.'

Philip's wife, Jean, had died from a rare form of brain cancer. One day she was well, the next she was admitted to hospital with double vision and a headache. The tumour was discovered on a CT scan the next day. Five months later she was dead. She had spent her last few precious months in hospital and for most of that time, Philip was by her side. Sometimes a kindly nurse would encourage him to go home and get some rest, promising that she would contact him if there was any change, but most of his time was spent in the hospital. He and Jean had met each other late in life and had no children. For the past ten years they had been inseparable. Now, she was gone.

'Thank you for telling me this,' I said. 'I can see it is not easy for you to talk about it, but I'm glad you did. You have a lot to feel sad about and I understand why you would want a way out, a break from it all.' I paused, aware that I could so easily silence him with a wrong word or gesture. That I could make him regret talking to me, if I appeared too upset or overwhelmed. He needed to know he could go on and that I would help him contain it, until he could manage by himself. He remained silent looking down at his hands. I decided to go on.

'Do you want to know what else I think?' I asked hesitantly, moving a little closer. He didn't pull back, but looked up expectantly for me to continue. 'I think it took a lot of courage to walk away from the edge of that platform. Even if you don't remember doing it. Some part of you has chosen to live. At least for now, some part of you says "yes" to life. Some part of you considers that you might have a future and is willing to take the risk.'

He didn't turn away. 'I'm not sure if that's what it is, Doctor, but I'm here anyway, however it happened,' he replied, quietly.

'Yes,' I said, 'you're here and I'm glad you came in.' There were no other words I could say. He was there in my consulting room and all I could do was be there with him, present with his suffering. In the background I could hear the waiting room murmurings, Bob Dylan's 'Forever Young' playing on the radio, the reception phone ringing, doors opening and closing, but in the consultation room there was only us and grief and the unanswerable questions. Is it worth it, the suffering and pain? Is there a limit to what one can be expected to bear? Is it wrong to think of ending it when that limit is reached? Philip wasn't the first to ask these questions and he would not be the last. Shakespeare's Hamlet had wrestled with the very same question when he had asked, 'Whether 'tis nobler in the mind to suffer the slings and arrows of outrageous fortune, or to take arms against a sea of troubles and by opposing, end them.' Albert Camus, a French philosopher, had considered suicide the only philosophical question worth asking. I still did not fully understand his answer, that 'it is only in accepting that the suffering of life is absurd and devoid of meaning that we can live and find meaning in this absurdity.' But this was not the time for the philosophical abstractions of Camus or Shakespeare. Not the time for religion with its teachings that God forbids suicide. I was neither poet, philosopher nor priest. Medicine was the path I had chosen. Medicine, with its manuals and protocols for dealing with all manner of diseases and illnesses, guidelines that trick us into thinking that there is an answer for everything, that we are in control. These manuals were lined up on my bookshelves, but nothing that I had read in them sprung to mind as being of use. I had no answers, no strategy or plan.

I looked away, his grief too exposed. The silence hung between us. I searched within my internal toolbox for something that might help. Almost involuntarily, I found myself taking deep but imperceptible breaths and silently repeating a meditation mantra on compassion that I had learned: 'May you live with ease. May you be free from suffering. May you be happy.' That was all I could do but at least, it stopped me distracting myself with my computer, fidgeting with my pen or handing out the tissues, as I sometimes did when faced with human suffering that took me way beyond my comfort zone. I remembered the first time I had met Philip, when he had come to see me almost twenty years earlier, when I'd first come to Killenaule. He had never attended a female doctor, he told me on our first encounter, sitting back in his seat, sizing me up. There was nothing suggestive about his scrutiny. It seemed to be to be an inner scrutiny, unconcerned with outward appearances. He needed to know if I was someone he could trust with his story, past, present and, possibly, future. He had the wisdom of a man who had suffered, a man who had lots of reasons to be wary of authority figures. I was aware that I was on trial, but had no idea what I needed to do to prove myself worthy of his trust.

Twenty years later, I was still there and he was still coming to see me. In the intervening years he had oscillated between darkness and light. It was because I had seen him in brighter times that I knew the depth of the darkness he was living with now and I feared for him. I knew what the guidelines advised. Risk assessment for suicide meant weighing the protective factors, such as strong religious belief and good social support, against the risk factors, such as isolation, previous psychiatric illness and alcohol or drug abuse. I knew that I should refer him to the Community Mental Health team, if I could not be sure of his safety. On paper, Philip met the high-risk criteria: he did not believe in God. His one close relationship had been severed. He had a previous history of depression. His one protective factor was that he did not have a problem with alcohol or drug abuse. I could not ensure his safety, but I knew Philip would not agree to meet with the Community Mental Health team. He had gone there previously, but said that he had not found the meetings helpful and had no wish ever to go back again. My presence was all that I had to offer him.

Philip caught me looking at the clock on my desk. He drew his jacket around him and began to zip it up. 'I'm sorry, Doctor,' he said, 'I have taken up a lot of your time. I'd better let you get on.'

He had been in for over twenty minutes, even though it had felt much shorter. It seemed petty to be concerned with time, considering the seriousness of what he had disclosed, but he was right, surgery must go on and it was up to me to bring the consultation to a satisfactory close. If I was a therapist, I would have said something like, 'OK, time to wrap up for today. I will see you at the same time next week and we can take it from there.' General practice does not work like that and wrapping up a consultation is sometimes the most difficult part. If I moved too fast, I could make Philip feel like I was abandoning or dismissing him; too slow, and I would never get to see the rest of the patients. I tentatively asked him if he would consider talking to someone like a bereavement counsellor. There were some counsellors who were not part of the mental health services and who were free for certain types of therapy.

He declined this offer. 'What good would that do?' he replied, looking up at me. 'I have said all I have to say to you. What would be the use in telling it all to someone who I never met before and who doesn't know anything about me? Look, I'll be OK. I just had a bad few days.'

He was zipping up his jacket as he spoke and I wondered if I had moved too fast. 'It's just a suggestion,' I said. 'I'm not saying you have to go, but they are there if you need them.'

'I know, Doctor,' he said, 'and thank you. I'm sorry I had to burden you with all that, but you know, if I told anybody else that I wanted to jump in front of a train, they would have me locked up.' He smiled briefly. 'You know they would, Doctor, and I really don't need that right now.'

'You're right,' I said, 'they probably would. But you know what it's like here, Philip. I don't have a whole lot of time to give you and I don't want you to think there is no one else. Bereavement counsellors can give you more time than I can and they can offer suggestions for coping with the pain that you are feeling.'

'Thanks, Doctor,' he said, 'but I actually feel better already. Don't worry, I won't do anything to harm myself. I have just had a bad few days. You know the way it is with me. Good days and bad days.'

I wasn't sure if he was trying to spare my feelings, or if he actually did feel better. I had to take him at face value. He had trusted me with his story. I had to trust him when he told me that he would not harm himself. He looked better, his face brighter and more like his usual self as he stood up to leave. It appeared as if he had regained a fraction of his equilibrium as he prepared to face the waiting room and what lay beyond.

As he left, I handed him a card with the number of a counsellor just in case he changed his mind. 'You were right to come in today,' I said, 'and I am glad you are feeling better. You know that I am here if you need me. But some day, I might not be here or you might need more than I can give you and if that happens, I would like to think that there is someone else that you can call, even if it is just to talk.'

'I'll have to think about it, Doctor. I'd better let you get on with your morning. Thanks again.' He left, with a nod and a thanks to Annemarie on the way out. I noticed that by then, the waiting room was full and a few people looked at their watches pointedly as he went out. I was well behind schedule but I was used to that.

I closed my door and sat quietly for a few seconds before I made my notes. 'Very low today,' my note read. 'Long discussion. Suicidal ideation, but no active intent at the moment. Declines referral, but may attend bereavement counselling. Feeling better when leaving.' That would have to cover it. A quick note on a computer could never convey the complexity of such a consultation. It was a paradox that the longer and more complex the consultation, the less time there was to record it. A couple of deep breaths later I opened the door again, stuck my head into the waiting room and called Mrs Brigid Hennessy, raising my voice to make sure I was heard over the din.

A few weeks later, I was waiting on the platform in Thurles for the Dublin train, my head bent over my phone, trying to find the email that told me the exact address of the meeting I was supposed to be attending that day.

'Well, good morning, Doctor,' I heard. 'Not in surgery today, I see.'

I looked up and saw that it was Philip, muffled up against the weather, rucksack on his back, making his way past me to the end of the platform. 'You'll have to move further down the platform if you want to get a seat,' he said. 'This train is always jammed. It stops at all the stops along the way.'

'Oh, thanks,' I replied. 'I should be OK, though, as I booked a seat last night.'

'Oh, you're alright then,' he replied, hesitating slightly, so that I couldn't help but ask him where he was off to. I wasn't being nosy, but he looked well and happy and to not ask would have seemed a bit odd. My interactions outside the surgery often seemed to be a delicate balance between displaying genuine interest and crossing a boundary that might be perceived as intrusive. I wondered if patients sometimes thought that I was always gathering information, that my questions had a medical agenda.

'I'm heading to England for a few days,' he said. 'A couple of my old friends from the building sites asked me over and I thought I might as well go.' He moved a bit closer and lowered his voice. 'I'm feeling much better,' he said. 'I rang that number you gave me and I went in a few times, just to talk. You were right. I did feel much better after it. I'll probably go back again when I get home.'

I was relieved. I had thought about Philip after he left the surgery that day and had felt the weight of responsibility for him. I had given Philip the number of the counsellor, as much for my benefit as his. I needed to share the burden. I needed him to have someone else. In reality, he could have harmed himself and how would I have felt about that? Who would believe me if I said that the reason that I did not send him to the mental health services was that he did not want to go? How would I have been judged for not insisting that he go? Sometimes, observing patient autonomy made things difficult. There was too much room for negotiation and compromise. If Philip had harmed himself, the investigation would have revealed that he had attended me in the previous week and that I had recorded his low mood, his suicidal ideation, but had not referred him to the specialists. While lots of well-meaning people have collated evidence to show that a high percentage of people who self-harm have attended their doctor in the previous few weeks or days, there is no information on the number of people who did not harm themselves following a helpful visit to their doctor. Thankfully, Philip did not come to any harm.

Just then we both heard the train. 'Well, I'd better get on,' he said, 'I'm hoping to get a seat.'

We boarded our separate carriages. Philip might well need my help someday, I thought, but for now he was back on track and even if I was the only one who had been aware of the depth of his despair, I also had the joy of knowing that he had overcome it, that his world was brighter again and that he was capable of travelling forward, while reconnecting with his past.

CHAPTER TWENTY-TWO

IRELAND'S FITTEST FAMILY

Ailshe's first WhatsApp message read:

'Hello family!
I probably should have said something at the weekend, but I may have entered us into Ireland's Fittest Family.'
(Three smiley faces) 12.06

Followed by the second one:

'And I just got an email and a voice message to ask if we are still interested???'
(Three horrified faces) 12.06

Followed by a third:

'I didn't think the application would come to anything.'
(One sad face) 12.06

Followed by a fourth:

They film it between May and August, I think.
(One smiley happy face.) 12.07

The responses were rapid and brief.

Joseph: *'Go on. Say we are and see what happens.'* 12.14

Liam Jnr: *'Yeah, fire away.'* 12.14

Liam Snr: *'That's a bit scary. But I suppose Mum or myself will be the passenger.'* 12.14

Ailshe: (who I presume had been sitting with her phone, holding her breath) *'Sorry, Mum. I thought I might be the strongest female, but feel free to say something?'*

(One laughing face.) 12.14

Me: *'Would LOVE to, but willing to sacrifice this opportunity to you, Ailshe, and promise not to sulk.'* 13.00

This was how the decision to enter the competition for the RTÉ television show *Ireland's Fittest Family* was made. There was no planning, no preparation, no training, no family conference, no mulling it over for days on end. Simply an eight-minute WhatsApp conversation, followed by an email from Ailshe to the organisers of the show, to say that the Meaghers were interested and would attend the fitness test. Hanging off bars over murky sea water, crawling through tunnels that looked like they could be rat-infested, jumping into ice-cold water, crawling along the ground, avoiding barbed wire, or carrying heavy weights up hundreds of steps, was not something I would consider fun, but they did not need me. The competition stipulated that the family team must consist of at least one parent and one female. They had the perfect combination and I, happily, left them to it.

The previous year, a Tipperary family had won the competition and the Meaghers figured they could make it two in a row for the county. Before long, Liam Snr began to doubt his sanity in agreeing to do it, however. Earlier in the year he had completed a triathlon and so considered himself relatively fit, but *Ireland's Fittest Family* required not only fitness but strength, competitiveness and mental toughness. 'I should never have done that triathlon,' he moaned. 'If I hadn't done that, Ailshe would never have considered entering us.'

But at that point, it was too late for regrets. The date for the fitness test was set and they were at least going to do that. Knowing there was no way out, Liam tried to convince me that it was my side of the family that had led to this mad streak in our children. I knew he meant my brothers, particularly the older two, Pat and Stephen, whose sanity was indeed questionable at times. On one occasion, Pat had been visiting Stephen in his home, the Old Monastery Hostel in Letterfrack. As Stephen served breakfast to the guests one man, an early riser, returned from his walk to say that he had spotted a man carrying what looked like a rowing machine up the Diamond Mountain.

'That will be my brother,' Stephen answered. 'He's always walking that rowing machine.'

The man, who was from Germany, turned to the guest beside him with a bewildered look and asked if it was an Irish custom to walk rowing machines. I have no way of verifying this story, but I do not doubt that Pat did actually carry the rowing machine from the hostel, along the trail in the Connemara National Park that ascends 440 metres to the summit of Diamond Hill. He then rowed a few kilometres at the top and carried it down again. A one-time Olympic rower, he was always setting himself challenges and I could certainly see that my children had inherited that tendency. But I wasn't about to take all the blame: there were questionable genes on both sides of the family. Liam's own brother, Paddy, had a large repertoire of adventure stories. His children, who had all miraculously reached adulthood unharmed, despite many skiing and boating near-misses, continued to accompany their father on trips, mainly to ensure his safety. His wife, Cathy, had long since given up bearing witness to such events. With such a mixture of genes, it was no wonder that our children were always looking for their next challenge, but I reassured Liam that they also had our caring genes, so that no matter what happened, they would not abandon him and would get him over the finish line, even if they had to carry him.

'You might well make little of it,' he said. 'You won't be the one making an idiot of yourself on television, in front of the nation.'

'No, I certainly will not,' I replied.

In the weeks that followed, the house and garden became a hive of activity. There was lifting, running, squatting, balancing, climbing, dangling and stretching, until finally the big day of the first event arrived. Once the competition began, there would be at least five rounds before the final. All of these were televised and while they were edited after the event, the competition did not allow for retakes. Once the starting signal sounded, there was no allowance for error.

Gradually, the news that the Meaghers were competing in *Ireland's Fittest Family* spread around Killenaule. They had been assigned Cork camogie legend Anna Geary as their coach, but were not allowed to tell anyone about this. Anna visited our home to assess their training schedule and to give them tips on managing the events. On the day she arrived, I left them to it and busied myself in the surgery. Later that evening, a patient asked me if it was true that Anna was their coach. I asked him what made him think that and he answered that a neighbour had heard roaring from the back garden in a voice that sounded suspiciously like Anna Geary's. I had to say I had no idea what he was talking about.

The filming finished in August and the show was not screened until November. During this time, some patients wanted to know if my family had got to the final. Others told me they had already heard that the Meaghers had won the competition, while others did not want any spoilers. They wanted the excitement of watching it on television. It appeared that this show was the highlight of the week for lots of families, after which the younger ones would go to bed and the older ones would set up their own obstacle courses in kitchens, sitting rooms and hallways all around the country and imagine they were in the show.

Excitement mounted leading up to the first episode, which featured six families battling it out to get to the next round. The Meaghers had got through only after competing in an elimination round, but they looked strong as Joseph hauled his father up onto a twelve-foot ramp, well ahead of the other team. Two weeks later, the second episode was screened. The first event included all four contestants carrying a heavy log between them, over rough terrain, dropping it and running through a muddy forest, picking it up again and finishing the competition. All four members of the team had to be in contact with the log before they could start running.

The Meaghers looked good at the start. Joseph led the team at the head of the log and they appeared to spring effortlessly along, but not long into this part of the event, it looked like Liam Jnr was in trouble. To an onlooker, he appeared to be staggering under the weight of the log. Their speed decreased and the other families passed them out. At six foot one, Liam Jnr was the tallest member of the family. He was also fit and strong from playing hurling and football, but at the end of that event he collapsed on the ground, gasping for breath. Beside him, Liam Snr was also lying flat out and gasping. But as the father recovered and the son did not, it became obvious that Liam Jnr had not just over-exerted himself but needed medical attention. His oxygen levels were surprisingly low, his blood pressure and pulse rate surprisingly high. He was pronounced unfit to proceed in the competition and an ambulance was arranged to bring him to hospital.

It was at that point of the actual, rather than the television, competition that I, sitting at home, keeping myself busy and trying not to think about their progress, got a call from Liam Snr.

He explained what had happened and asked if I could make my way to hospital to be with Liam Jnr. If anyone was to be weak and sick after an event, I had expected it to be Liam Snr, not this tall, healthy, vibrant, fit 19-year-old, who had left the house in high spirits the previous evening. I could tell that his father was worried about him, but he had to stay and complete the competition, as they would now have to compete in the elimination round without Liam Jnr.

I was concerned as I made my way to the hospital. Liam Jnr had played sport all his life and had never had any health problems, but my biggest worry was that he had suffered a cardiac arrhythmia, an abnormal heart rhythm brought on by exercise, which could have been fatal. However, I was not one to panic and assumed that whatever it was, he would recover.

When I got to the hospital, Liam Jnr was lying on a trolley, still in his wet and muddy sports gear, vomiting into a hospital receptacle. It took me some time to find someone who could give me any update on his diagnosis or what they could do for him. After a few hours, it was clear that his heart was not the cause of the collapse, but that he had suffered an abnormally high rise in an enzyme called creatine phosphokinase (CPK) that was probably due to a combination of carrying the heavy log, causing muscle injury to his neck, and the extreme exertion. He needed rehydration and rest in order to bring this enzyme back to normal levels, otherwise he was at risk of renal damage. The doctor wanted to keep him in hospital overnight for observation and he was advised not to even think about taking part in sport or exercise until his blood tests were normal and this could take a minimum of three weeks. I could live with this, even if Liam Jnr began to protest as the IV fluids helped him feel better.

I conveyed all of this to his father, who, I knew, would be concerned and who still had to compete in another round of the competition. The eliminator round consisted of running and jumping and crawling through mud. The final task required that all three family members get to the top of a ten-foot wall. Joseph was first up, followed by Ailshe, with his help. The Meaghers were leading. They only needed to get Liam Snr over the wall to win and qualify for the next round. Liam ran at the wall, reached for Joseph's hand, but narrowly missed it and slid back down to the bottom. He made another attempt. He ran, jumped up, and managed to catch Joseph's hand, but did not have the strength to haul himself up and let go and slid to the bottom again. He repeated this a few more times, until the final whistle sounded and they realised all three of the competing team were already over their wall. The show was over. The cameras faded and that was it. The end of the road for the Meaghers.

In the hospital, Liam Jnr kept checking his phone and asking me it there was any news on the competition results. He wasn't very hopeful as he was aware that that the other teams would put their best people forward, while his team was missing him, a key component of their strategy for getting up ramps and over high walls. Eventually, the disappointing news reached us. I reassured him that he had done well to finish the first event, considering that he was now in a hospital, connected to IV fluids.

When the others arrived to see him that evening, the mood was glum and sombre, because they had been knocked out of the competition, but all three were relieved to see Liam Jnr sitting up in bed, insisting that he was well enough to go home.

'That bloody wall,' Liam Snr kept repeating. 'I almost had it. I just didn't have anything left in the tank.'

'Look, Dad,' Joseph said. 'You didn't even get to eat or get dry between events, because you were waiting with Liam for the ambulance to come. You did extraordinarily well, considering everything.'

'Oh, I know, but I will be haunted forever more by that bloody wall. I don't know how I will bear to watch it on TV. It's just so disappointing, because we were doing so well.'

'I know,' Joseph said, clearly disappointed, but trying to hide it. He turned to his sister and put his arm around her shoulder. 'It has been great fun and thank you, Ailshe, for entering us into it. Even though we lost, I have really enjoyed it. I would do it all over again.'

'I'll keep in touch with the organisers,' Ailshe said, surprisingly sanguine and accepting of their situation. 'As soon as next year's applications come out, I'll let ye know.'

I looked at Liam Jnr, who was still pale and weak and tired, despite his protestations that he did not need to be in hospital. 'Steady on, Ailshe,' he said. 'Not so fast. At least let me get out of hospital.'

The Monday morning after the screening of that episode, Liam and I were both in the surgery, but it was impossible to get through consultations in any sort of timely manner, as everybody wanted to discuss *Ireland's Fittest Family*. Before half-past nine, Annemarie had already answered the phone to at least five callers, who wanted to pass on their congratulations to Dr. Meagher and his family on their television appearance. Nobody seemed to notice that they had just been eliminated. Everybody wanted to commend them on their effort. One man commented that Dr Meagher was marvellous to be in surgery, back at work so soon, as he thought the competition had taken place in real time, the evening before. I explained that it had been recorded a few months earlier and that they were all well recovered by then, but I don't think he really understood how that worked. It seemed like everybody had seen it and everybody had an opinion.

A few months later, when the excitement had almost completely died down, Brigid, a woman in her early seventies, shared her experience of watching the show with me. 'Your family!' she exclaimed. 'On the television! I thought I would have a heart attack. I could hardly bear to watch it. I had to ask my husband what was going on and he couldn't answer me, because he was shouting so much at the television.'

We chatted about the show, about how Liam Jnr was fully recovered and how much enjoyment they had got out of doing it, until I managed to steer the consultation back to medical matters. 'Two things, Doctor Gannon,' she said, when I suggested we had better get back to business. 'I need my prescription and I wonder if you would mind signing this form for me? I'm going to Lourdes with the diocese and I need you to say that I am well enough to go. I hate bothering you with a form, but I have to send this in if I want to get a place.'

'It's no bother,' I said, as I reached out to take it from her and filled in the required information. I went through her prescription, double-checking that she had everything she needed on it, looked at her file to see if her bloods and blood pressure measurements were up to date and made sure there was nothing outstanding, or that I was neglecting to follow up. Everything seemed to be in order, so I quickly printed the script and handed it to her with the signed form, reminding her to call to Annemarie on the way out to get it stamped.

She rose, put on her coat and made her way towards the door. 'I know there is a charge for forms,' she said, 'so, I'll give the money to Annemarie.'

'Look, we'll let that one go,' I said. 'You might say a prayer for me when you are in Lourdes and that will cover it.'

'Thanks, Doctor Gannon. I would do that anyway, but I'll do better than that. I will bring you back a bottle of holy water.'

'Thanks very much, Bridget,' I replied, 'that's very thoughtful, but I'm sure you have enough people to think about when you are there, besides me.'

'It's not for you at all, Doctor Gannon,' she said, without hesitation. 'It's so you can throw it over Doctor Meagher, and maybe he will be able to get himself over the wall next time.'

CHAPTER TWENTY-THREE

A TIME TO REMEMBER

Although it was not yet midday, the sun was high in a clear blue cloudless sky. The pale pink blossoms of the apple trees littered the path to the clothesline and beyond. Both dogs, Dax, our giant black Labrador retriever, and Shad, a small Yorkshire terrier, who had come to us by accident, followed me into the garden. I kept one eye on Dax, who was liable to bolt over what had once been a miniature football pitch for the children to visit his friend Tao, Judith's mature, mild-mannered husky, who lived a couple of fields away. But the day was too hot for running. Dax stretched himself out full-length on the grass, panting, while Shad stood at the entrance to a rabbit hole, growling at whatever danger he imagined lurked there. The football pitch was silent. The goalposts stood tall and erect at either end and as I stood in the stillness of the morning, I could have sworn that I heard the ding of a sliotar hitting the crossbar, followed by a whoop of delight at another goal saved. But I was just imagining it. There were no children's cries. There were no longer any bruised knees or scratched elbows to attend to. Dax and Shad were my only companions as I hung the washing on the line.

I had returned the previous night from a week away with college friends, an annual event since our children had grown and become independent. I looked forward to these holidays for months before I went and continued to savour them for months after I came home. It was a week of reconnection, a time to remember who I had been before becoming a wife, mother and doctor. A time to reconnect with the insecure, self-critical medical student, who had no idea what the future held, but who liked to appear as if she did. In the company of my friends I could let that person resurface and merge with the one I had become: a little more tolerant, a little more accepting, a lot more at ease in the world, with the same, if not more, capacity for joy. In the intervening years, all of us had had our share of joys, sorrows, losses and disappointments, but within a short time of being back together, we could still finish each other's sentences, laugh at our differences and cherish our history.

On the outward journey, we'd boarded the plane and sat in our separate seats. As I'd settled into my book, the lady next to me had touched me lightly on the shoulder. 'I think your friend is trying to get your attention,' she said.

I looked up to see my friend, Íde, gesticulating unselfconsciously at the top of the plane, indicating that there was an empty seat beside her. I moved to sit in the seat, while she gazed out of the window, picking out the landmarks below. Within a few minutes, a man sat down in the unoccupied aisle seat next to me, asking if we would mind, as he'd felt a bit squashed in the seat he was in further back. I suspected he had noticed Íde's gesticulations and thought that she would be good company on an otherwise uneventful journey.

As we chatted, he asked how long we had been friends. 'Since 1980,' I said, 'almost forty years.'

He let out a low whistle. 'That's something to celebrate', he replied. 'A lot of history there, I would say.'

It was a long time to be friends, I realised, wondering if the shared experiences of medical training had bound us together. Throughout my six years in college, my classmates had become more like a large extended family than friends. Despite our living apart and leading busy lives, the bonds we formed then would have been more difficult to undo than to maintain.

Now, I put the empty laundry basket down and looked around the garden, reluctant to leave the warm sunshine to go back into the shade of the house. The wild flowers that I had planted a few years earlier consisted now of only a few forlorn, eponymous forget-me-nots, which bloomed year after year without attention. When I had planted them, I had assumed that 'wild flowers' meant that they would look after themselves and was very disappointed to find that like most things which provide joy, all but the forget-me-nots needed regular attention, if they were to survive. Further along the bank a small crop of bluebells, a gift from the garden of an elderly patient, were going to seed. I picked some and automatically sniffed them. Before going away, I'd barely registered that they were there. The ash tree planted in memory of my grandmother many years earlier stood tall and straight, its branches already covered in leaves. I pulled a battered garden chair from its abandoned location beside the shed, placed it under the tree and sat on it. I closed my eyes and imagined my grandmother's face: soft skin, gold-rimmed glasses framing her blue eyes and the dimples that so many of us had inherited. Here, under this tree, I could feel her presence and knew she would be proud of Liam and me and her great-grandchildren and what we had achieved.

Dax joined me under the tree. 'What do you think, Dax?' I asked him, rubbing his head. 'Do you think GranGran can see us now?' He looked at me as if to say that I was the most interesting and intelligent person in the world. He seemed to be thanking me for coming back from wherever it was I had to go, while at the same time, pleading with me not to go away again. I looked up and saw the swallows, flying higher than I have ever seen them fly. Every year, they returned to their nests under the eaves. Perhaps they'd been there before I left, but I did not notice them. I stayed a while in the shade of the tree, enjoying this, the last day of my holidays.

Joseph had, by then, moved to the UK to study statistics. He would, all going to plan, eventually be Joseph Meagher PhD, a doctor of numbers, rather than humans. He was very good at keeping in touch and his phone calls could go on for quite a while. I seemed to have fallen into the role of counsellor and advisor on all matters related to work–life balance, relationships, goal-setting and the general meaning of life. Liam Snr discussed politics in general with him, Brexit in particular and all things related to GAA. I was glad to know that I had not ended Joseph's GAA career by sending him to Ring and he was still very involved in hurling and football in the UK. Ailshe and Liam Jnr took turns providing him with all the other news.

During one of our conversations, I had asked Joseph how he would feel if we moved away from Killenaule. I wondered if he would miss it. Joseph was used to the hypothetical questions that I sometimes posed, often just as a means of keeping him a bit longer on the phone. 'What are the chances of ye actually moving?' he asked, I presume trying to gauge how much effort he needed to put into his reply, but also because I think his brain now thought in probabilities.

'Zero,' I replied. 'I'm just wondering if you have any thoughts on it.'

'Well, I would certainly miss the hurling pitch. A lot of my memories are of matches and training sessions and the lads I played with. I would definitely miss that. But I think I would miss Jimmy and Mary most.'

Joseph had first started visiting our neighbours, Jimmy and Mary Ryan, as a young boy of nine or ten. Jimmy was a well-known hurley-maker and we were privileged to have him and his workshop right next door. Joseph would visit him in the workshop, where Jimmy, covered from head to toe in sawdust, would regale him with all sorts of stories that Joseph never tired of hearing. From there, he would go to the yard to play with their dog, a small Lakeland terrier called Bruno, before progressing to the kitchen, where Mary would feed him freshly baked scones. Joseph reminded me of the day that he had been so involved in playing with Bruno that he had stepped back and fallen straight into their pond. Jimmy, hearing the splash, had appeared out of his workshop, just in time to see Joseph struggling to his feet, his clothes and shoes dripping wet. 'Check your pockets before you go,' he'd said. 'Make sure you're not taking any of my fish home with you.' Joseph had dutifully begun to check his pockets before realising that, once again, Jimmy had caught him out.

When I rang Joseph recently to say that Jimmy had passed away at the age of 90, he mourned the loss of his childhood friend. To Joseph, Jimmy had always been a friend, never an old man, and Mary and Jimmy's house and workshop had had a large part to play in making Killenaule his home.

Liam Jnr never had any trouble feeling at home in Killenaule, returning from college each weekend and holiday with a full itinerary of sporting and social events, leaving the hallway strewn with hurleys, smelly gear bags and muddy football boots. His older brother and sister frequently admonished me for being too soft on him, for not insisting that he maintain a bit more order in his surroundings – but although I valued order, I also knew that his days in our house and his summers in Killenaule were numbered and I probably treasured them more than he did. Besides, since I'd discovered Marie Kondo's *The Life-Changing*

Magic of Tidying Up, my house, apart from the hallway and Liam's bedroom, was a model of organisation and neatness. With the enthusiasm with which I embraced many an 'improvement project', I had divested myself of anything that did not 'spark joy' and had organised everything else into neatly folded, colour-coded rows, in cupboards and drawers. The hot press contained neat stacks of 'bed bundles', matching bed linen tied with brightly coloured ribbons, and sometimes when I went there to retrieve a set of clean bed linen, I stopped to survey the orderly bundles, just to remind myself of how far I had come since the days when I did not know where anything was – in that cupboard or, indeed, in the chaotic life I had led, balancing and juggling family and work. Nowadays, I could handle a few wayward hurleys and football boots. Nowadays, I was more aware of what sparked joy and one of those things, or people, would be leaving home for good soon enough. Before long, I would hear the sound of posters being taken off his bedroom wall as he prepared to make his nest elsewhere and I would miss him when he was gone.

Summer flew quickly by, as I knew it would, and before I knew it, the swallows had left. It seemed like such a short time ago that I had sat under the ash tree watching their antics. Liam Jnr had also returned to college in Cork where he was studying engineering.

'Do you think I should apply for the GP Training Scheme?' Ailshe asked me one day. I realised, with a start, that it was already late October and that the application forms for GP training had just been posted online. Ailshe had qualified as a doctor that summer and had just completed the first three months of her internship in Dublin. I had never encouraged her to consider becoming a GP, but I had never discouraged her either. Her career choices were endless: medicine, surgery, paediatrics, psychiatry, public health, microbiology, pathology, radiology, emergency care and general practice were only some of the choices on offer.

'Do you think you would like general practice?' I asked, a little surprised that she would contemplate such a career, considering all the dinner-table stories she had heard down through the years, coupled with reports of how Irish general practice was struggling to retain doctors, due to emigration, retirement and lack of government funding. I was secretly pleased, however, not that she was thinking of doing general practice, but that she was not thinking of joining so many young doctors who were leaving for Australia, New Zealand or Canada after their internship. Ailshe's long-term boyfriend, Brendan, who had qualified as an engineer at the same time as Ailshe, had taken up a two-year job commitment in Kilkenny and if this was Ailshe's rationale for staying, then it was yet another reason for me to be grateful that this young man had come into our lives and was, by now, practically part of the family.

'I think I would,' she replied. 'I am just not sure if I should do a hospital specialty first and then apply for a GP Scheme, or go straight into general practice.'

'But why do you think you would like being a GP?' I asked. She laughed and said that if I could do it, then she figured anybody could. I advised her to consider the possibility that perhaps I had a knack of making things look easy and to prepare for a rude awakening if she did choose general practice.

'Of course, I'm only teasing you,' she said. 'I just think that I could be good at it. I certainly know a lot about it and I know even though you and Dad worked a lot when we were young, I always felt that you were here when we needed you and if you weren't here, you were just at the bottom of the drive and I knew where to find you.'

I had forgotten that the decision to build the surgery and house on the same site was so that Liam and I would be close to home, if we were needed. That had been important to us at the time, but I had not thought that my children had been aware of, or valued, that proximity.

'But what about the work?' I asked. 'All those stories you have heard from Dad and me when you were younger. All those things that you said would drive you mad?'

'Well, I certainly would not tolerate the man who complained about sweating too much, but didn't think to take off one of the ten layers he was wearing while sitting in the waiting room. I think I would have sent him packing pretty swiftly. Or the woman who said that the consultant had not put her off the cigarettes and so she thought that meant she should continue smoking. Or all the people who won't take the flu injection, because they say it gave them the flu more than twenty years ago.'

I had grown used to people's idiosyncrasies, to the myths, half-truths, certainties and sometimes daft things that some people said to me on an almost daily basis. I had developed a well-tuned filter that was constantly working unobtrusively to only register the signal: I had become much better at disregarding the noise. Every day, I treated people who did not take their medication because they had read in the paper that it was bad for them, or people who took an alternative therapy because they had read on the internet that it was good for them. All I could do was to advise people based on the scientific evidence of the time. I could not know what was going to be proved right or wrong in the future. Over the years, I had worked according to guidelines, only to find that a few years later, these guidelines were altered and a few years later they were altered again. But I tried, at least, to be honest about the limitations of science and the dynamic nature of evidence. I consoled myself with the words of Dara Ó Briain: 'Science knows it doesn't know everything. Otherwise, it'd stop'.

However, I had grown less tolerant of quackery and fully agree with Ó Briain when he disputes the notion that everyone's opinion is equally valid; that just because science does not have all the answers, it does not mean that anyone and everyone can fill in the gaps with nonsense; that if someone wants to see a 'toothiologist' rather than a dentist for their dental problems and follow the advice of a 'nutritionist' instead of a dietitian for digestive problems, I might not be able to do anything about it, but I certainly did not have to condone it.

'You will have no problem dealing with the patients,' I said to Ailshe, knowing how sociable and interested in people she was. 'You are more likely to be frustrated by the volume of workload and the limited resources available to GPs. But I wouldn't let that put you off. When your father and I returned from the UK many years ago and made plans to build a surgery in a field, many people told us we were mad.' I had no regrets about that decision. I believed that Liam and I had made a difference to people's health and well-being. There might not be any way to measure those effects, but life is not a clinical trial and as Albert Einstein is once said to have written on a blackboard: 'Not everything that can be counted counts and not everything that counts can be counted.'

I thought about some of those unquantifiable outcomes, the unseen effects of having an accessible, affordable and skilful family doctor: unwanted pregnancies could be avoided by providing contraception; possible suicides could be prevented by being there to listen and refer; strokes, heart attacks and limb amputations reduced, by managing diabetes and high blood pressure. Most of all, I thought of the number of people who had been treated at home during their final illness, because that had been their wish. It doesn't matter how much more advanced medicine becomes, people are always going to get sick and die and when the hospitals cannot do any more, most people wish for a trusted, skilful, knowledgeable doctor to facilitate this in the comfort of their home, surrounded by their family and friends.

'I'm still not sure, Mum,' Ailshe said. The applications are already LIVE and so I have to decide in the next week or so.'

As always, that would be her own decision. I had no doubt that whatever she chose, she would do the best she could, and no one could expect any more than that. 'You know,' I said. 'It's only a job at the end of the day, like any other. You have your degree and so there are so many doors open to you.' I thought that her path would unfold and probably change direction a few times, bringing her to places that she had not planned to go. At her age, I had no idea of the many different paths that I would travel. I had certainly never planned to write a book. I added that I thought it best to set goals, but hold them lightly and celebrate all the successes along the way; sometimes, making progress towards your goal is more rewarding than actually achieving it.

During this conversation Liam Snr had been sitting across the table from us, putting together a giant-sized, home-cooked-ham sandwich that he proceeded to eat with relish. He was wearing a blue shirt, the colour of his eyes, open at the neck, without a tie. Ever since the scientific literature had suggested that doctors' ties could be a source of infection, Liam had happily abandoned his, although he still would not let me get rid of any from the collection he had amassed over the years, no matter how much I extolled the virtues of Marie Kondo and the benefits of a decluttered home. Looking at him across the table, I saw again the young man I had fallen in love with. The young man whose dance moves had caught my eye in the Oasis nightclub in Salthill on one of our class nights out. I remembered how, from then on, my heart would quicken when I saw his red bicycle in the bicycle rack on my way into the hospital, or his long, blue woollen scarf hanging in the cloakroom. But I played cool, too cool, until one night after we qualified, realising that it might be my last chance, I ran after him as he left a party and asked him if he would walk me home. He did. And the rest, as they say, is history.

Liam caught me looking at him. 'I bet you're thinking that I am the most wonderful husband in the world,' he said.

'For once, you're absolutely right,' I replied, but I don't think he believed me.

Outside the kitchen window, the late October leaves were floating to the ground, like snowflakes heralding a snowstorm. A feeling I have come to recognise as gratitude crept over me. It began somewhere in my chest and spread outwards, creating a cocoon of warmth, ease and joy. The words my daughter had said, 'You were always here when we needed you', made me realise how fortunate I had been. Combining motherhood and career had never been easy and many times over the years I had worried that I was not managing either as well as I should, but I had done my best and Ailshe, with her casual observation, had made me realise that my best had probably been good enough.

'What's the matter, Mum?' Ailshe asked. 'You have gone all quiet and you look a bit sad.'

'Not sad, sweetie,' I said, smiling and rising to give her a hug. 'Not a bit sad. Just grateful for all that I have and all that is yet to come.'

Susan McKay is an award-winning Irish journalist and the author of two critically acclaimed books, *Sophia's Story* (Gill and Macmillan) and *Northern Protestants: An Unsettled People* (Blackstaff Press).

'This is a most important book because we must remember and it is too easy to forget. Susan McKay has handled grief and anger with great clearheadedness. In spite of the horror in this book, it is very hard to put it aside.' Jennifer Johnstone

'One of the most invaluable, heart-wrenching, and poignant insights into the sheer wickedness, and the human catastrophe, of the Troubles.' Kevin Myers, *Irish Independent*

'A necessary book, which restores humanity to those among the dead who tend to be remembered in terms of statistics alone. Susan McKay has gone about her difficult task with bravery and finesse.' Patricia Craig, *Independent*

'Tremendously moving . . . Anyone who wants to understand the sectarian conflict of Northern Ireland must examine the individual tragedies that go to make up the broader narrative. This is the grim task to which McKay so admirably applies herself . . . These fine books form part of a more noble cause, what Milan Kundera called the struggle of memory against forgetting.' Andrew Anthony, *Observer*

'Peace can only endure if the dead can finally be laid to rest. *Bear in Mind These Dead* is a moving and important contribution to that process.' *Derry Journal*

'Susan McKay is a writer and journalist of courage, integrity and humanity . . . it is salutary to have a vivid reminder of the sheer awfulness of the slaughter . . . ensuring that the dead are not forgotten is done sensitively and objectively without any voyeurism or sensationalism . . . Susan McKay has produced another fine book of lasting value.' Martin Mansergh, *Village Magazine*